SOCIOLOGICAL PERSPECTIVES ON HEALTH, ILLNESS AND HEALTH CARE

SOCIOLOGICAL PERSPECTIVES ON HEALTH, ILLNESS AND HEALTH CARE

Edited by

David Field *BA, MA, AM, PhD*
Deputy Director
Centre for Cancer and Palliative Care Studies,
Institute of Cancer Research/Royal Marsden NHS Trust

Steve Taylor *BA, LLB, MPhil, PhD*
Lecturer in Medical Sociology
King's College, London,
London School of Economics and
Coventry University

**Blackwell
Science**

© 1998 by
Blackwell Science Ltd
Editorial Offices:
Osney Mead, Oxford OX2 0EL
25 John Street, London WC1N 2BL
23 Ainslie Place, Edinburgh EH3 6AJ
350 Main Street, Malden
    MA 02148 5018, USA
54 University Street, Carlton
    Victoria 3053, Australia
10, rue Casimir Delavigne
    75006 Paris, France

Other Editorial Offices:

Blackwell Wissenschafts-Verlag GmbH
Kurfürstendamm 57
10707 Berlin, Germany

Blackwell Science KK
MG Kodenmacho Building
7–10 Kodenmacho Nihombashi
Chuo-ku, Tokyo 104, Japan

First published 1998

Set in 10/12.5 Century Book
by DP Photosetting, Aylesbury, Bucks
Printed and bound in Great Britain by
MPG Books Ltd, Bodmin, Cornwall

The Blackwell Science logo is a
trade mark of Blackwell Science Ltd,
registered at the United Kingdom
Trade Marks Registry

DISTRIBUTORS

Marston Book Services Ltd
PO Box 269
Abingdon
Oxon OX14 4YN
(*Orders:* Tel: 01235 465500
          Fax: 01235 465555)

USA
Blackwell Science, Inc.
Commerce Place
350 Main Street
Malden, MA 02148 5018
(*Orders:* Tel: 800 759 6102
          781 388 8250
          Fax: 781 388 8255)

Canada
Login Brothers Book Company
324 Saulteaux Crescent
Winnipeg, Manitoba R3J 3T2
(*Orders:* Tel: 204 224-4068)

Australia
Blackwell Science Pty Ltd
54 University Street
Carlton, Victoria 3053
(*Orders:* Tel: 03 9347 0300
          Fax: 03 9347 5001)

A catalogue record for this title
is available from the British Library

ISBN 0-632-04147-1

Library of Congress
Cataloging-in-Publication Data

Sociological perspectives on health, illness
    and health care/edited by David Field,
    Steve Taylor.
        p.   cm.
    Includes bibliographical references
    and index.
    ISBN 0-632-04147-1 (pbk.)
    1. Social medicine.   I. Field, David,
    1942– .   II. Taylor, Steve (Steve D.)
    RA418.S67337   1998
    306.4′61–dc21   97-39128
                                        CIP

Contents

List of Contributors

Ellen Annandale, *BSc, MA, PhD,* Lecturer, Department of Sociology, University of Warwick

Sara Arber, *BSc, MSc, PhD,* Professor of Sociology, University of Surrey

Rob Baggott, Reader in Public Policy, Department of Public Policy and Managerial Studies, De Montfort University, Leicester,

Mel Bartley, *MA, MSc, PhD,* Principal Research Fellow, Department of Epidemiology and Public Health, University College London

David Blane, *MB, BS, MSc,* Lecturer in Sociology Applied to Medicine, Charing Cross and Westminster Medical School

Mary Boulton, *BA, PhD,* Senior Lecturer in Sociology as Applied to Medicine, Imperial College School of Medicine

George Davey Smith, *BA, MBBChir, MA, MSc, MD, MFPHM,* Professor of Clinical Epidemiology, Department of Social Medicine, University of Bristol

David Field, *BA, MA, AM, PhD,* Deputy Director, Centre for Cancer and Palliative Care Studies, Institute of Cancer Research/Royal Marsden NHS Trust

Ray Fitzpatrick, *BA, MSc, PhD,* Professor of Public Health and Primary Care, University of Oxford

Jay Ginn, *BSc, MSc, PhD,* Research Fellow, Department of Sociology, University of Surrey

Graham Hart, *BA, PhD,* Deputy Director, MRC Medical Sociology Research Unit, Glasgow

Allison James, *BA, PhD,* Lecturer in Applied Anthropology, Department of Sociology and Anthropology, Hull University

Veronica James, *RGN, MA, PhD,* Professor of Nursing, University of Nottingham

Mike Kelly, *BA, MPhil, PhD,* Professor of Social Sciences, University of Greenwich

Lindsay Prior, *BSc, MA, PhD,* Senior Lecturer in Social Research Methods, School of Social and Administrative Studies, University of Wales, Cardiff

Mike Saks, *BA, MA, PhD,* Professor and Dean of the Faculty of Health and Community Sciences, De Montfort University, Leicester

Steve Taylor, *BA, LLB, MPhil, PhD,* Lecturer in Medical Sociology, King's College London, London School of Economics and Coventry University

Nick Tilley, *BSc, MSc,* Professor of Sociology, Crime and Social Research Unit, Nottingham Trent University

Acknowledgements

The manuscript for this book was mainly assembled by David Field while he was working in the Department of Sociology at the University of Plymouth. David would like to acknowledge the department's practical support for this work and the personal benefits of working in its friendly and collegial environment.

Tables 2.1 and 11.2 are published with permission of the Office for National Statistics, and tables 7.1 and 7.2 with permission of the Health Education Authority and the ONS. Other tables are based on Crown copyright statistics.

Introduction

David Field and Steve Taylor

The study of health, illness and health care continues to be a major area of sociological activity as can be seen by the continuing stream of new books and articles in specialist and general sociological journals and in those of the health professions and para-professions. The Medical Sociology Group is the largest study group of the British Sociological Association, attracting over 300 participants to its annual conference. Sociology of health and illness courses have become increasingly popular options on undergraduate courses in the social sciences and have become mandatory for a growing number of health practitioners at diploma, undergraduate and Master's level. However, although broader sociological concerns may be used to inform the discussion of particular issues, attempts to integrate the general concerns of the broader discipline with the specific concerns of the sub-discipline are comparatively rare and dated (Friedson 1988, first published 1970; Gerhardt 1989, Scambler 1987). The notable exception is Bury (1997) who draws upon current sociological concerns to develop a sustained and critical theoretical argument about health and illness in contemporary society. Introductory texts for undergraduate sociology students (e.g. Nettleton 1996, Turner 1995) and medical, nursing and other health students (e.g. Bond & Bond 1994, Scambler 1994, Taylor & Field 1997) variously draw upon current conceptual issues, such as 'post-modernism', Foucaldian approaches and the role of the body but, by their very nature, are unable to provide the level of analysis suitable for students and practitioners who already possess a working knowledge of sociology.

This book developed from our concern about lack of readily available general 'post-introductory' level sources for use in our teaching of the sociology of health and illness and attempts to go some way towards correcting this situation. It aims to reflect the range and diversity of sociological approaches to the study of health and illness in contemporary Britain and to provide up-to-date and in-depth examinations of key issues and topics within the area. To this end sociologists with an established record of research were invited to contribute original essays on their area of expertise and asked to give their interpretations of the current state of knowledge in their area, and to identify key issues and emerging directions in research. It should be stressed that this is not an introductory text as it is neither an introduction to the subject nor does it aim to be comprehensive. Rather, it assumes knowledge and familiarity with sociological terms and concepts and attempts to build upon and take forward issues raised and addressed by sociologists working in the area. We hope that the chapters will not only inform readers of current developments in research and conceptualisation but that they will also encourage and enable readers to analyse and question these in a critical manner.

Part I of the book is concerned with problems of conceptualisation and research. In Chapter 1, Kelly and Field suggest that sociological conceptualisations of chronic illness as inevitably disruptive of, and separate from, the 'normal' world of everyday life reflect the assumptions which sociologists have made about the nature of modern western industrial societies. They suggest that these have more to do with the social structuring of the experience of chronic illness by such societies than with any 'inevitable' consequences of chronic illness. In contemporary Britain such conceptualisations are now being challenged as inadequately describing the experience of chronic illness and disability. Kelly and Field suggest new conceptualisations are required which take account of the more fragmented and 'open' social structuring of everyday life and the greater variety of ways in which chronic illness may be experienced.

Another area of contemporary contention and concern is mental illness, reflected in its most extreme form in mass media depictions of the failures of community care for people who are mentally ill. In his chapter Prior considers practical and conceptual problems in the ways in which psychiatric cases are defined and constructed. He argues that such problems are practically resolved by psychiatric and other health and social workers in terms of organisational requirements rather than in terms of 'intrinsic' properties of psychiatric symptoms or the needs of clients. That this may result in the person disappearing from the view of helping agencies is illustrated by reference to two well-publicised and tragic case histories.

It is a sociological truism that facts do not speak for themselves, but have to be organised and interpreted within theoretical concepts of one sort or another. Thus, the very process of doing social research – whether acknowledged or not by the researcher – necessarily involves making theoretical assumptions about the nature of the social world and how it is to be understood. These assumptions inevitably influence how research problems are conceptualised, what is 'found' and how such 'findings' are interpreted. Taylor and Tilley examine the relationship between theory and method in the sociological interview. They suggest that traditional structured and unstructured interview methods both share a common assumption that it is the respondent who is the subject of an interview. Arguing from a scientific realist position they suggest that the subject of a sociological interview is, in fact, the researcher's theory. The implications of this idea are illustrated with data from 'realist interviews' with anorectic children.

Sociologists are often called upon to provide research evidence to inform decisions about health issues of practical concern. Hence, much of the research in the sociology of health and illness is 'applied' and driven by the requirements of policy. The final chapter in this section turns to some of the practical problems of conducting policy oriented research in a sensitive area. Boulton, Fitzpatrick and Hart discuss the issues they confronted in a ten-year programme of research into the sexual behaviour of homosexual and bi-sexual men in relation to HIV/ AIDS, indicating the different ways in which sociology can contribute to public health through the definition of issues which should be addressed and the choice of sociological methods to do so. One of the aims of their research was to provide accurate descriptions of such behaviour with a view to informing the development of social policy. This raises important issues of the reliability and validity of the data collected, especially given the sensitive nature of the topic. Boulton *et al.* attempted to solve this by using both quantitative and qualitative methods, which they discuss in some detail. They also discuss the difficulties of recruiting gay males and talking openly about sexual behaviour with them.

The second section of the book reflects the enduring sociological interest in social divisions within society. Within sociology, social class has been a major concept for explaining inequality and deprivation and the distribution of life chances within society. Blane, Bartley and Davey Smith provide a critical review of the substantial body of research material on socio-economic factors and health produced since the publication of the influential Black Report on *Inequalities in Health* (Townsend *et al.* 1988). An appreciation of how 'social class' and 'health' are measured is central to any evaluation of this research evidence, so the first part of the chapter addresses these methodological issues. Blane *et al.* go on to suggest that three pathways can be identified between socio-economic factors and health and argue that the relationship between them can be best understood within a life course perspective.

Most of the sociological research on childhood illness has focused upon the effect of such illness upon the family, the disability of children, and how these are managed by adults. The experiences of the children themselves scarcely figure in this research. In Chapter 6 James suggests this is a result of the contemporary Western view of childhood which constructs children as incompetent, vulnerable and dependent upon adults. Even where the impact of illness upon the child is the focus of research interest, their experiences are solicited at second-hand from parents and other adults involved in their care and the child's role in making sense of their illness experience is often ignored. Ethnographic studies have shown that children are competent role performers who can recognise and manage competing social and cultural interpretations and expectations of their sick roles. James argues that sociological approaches to health and illness in children must recognise the active role of the child and acknowledge the rights of sick children.

Sociologists now recognise that gender is a fundamentally important social division – a recognition which is the result of feminist research and writing. Annandale, in Chapter 7, notes that both feminist theory and the sociology of health and illness contest the bio-medical model and seek to develop theoretical approaches based upon social rather than upon 'natural' or biological explanations of health and illness. Her project is to 'reintegrate feminist theory into the sociology of health and illness'. The chapter therefore explores interpretations of the relationship between gender and health status from different theoretical feminist perspectives. She examines the post-modern critique of liberal and radical feminist agendas, looking at both its theoretical potential to inform gender differences in health status and the political dangers of the deconstruction of gender in contemporary patriarchal society.

In contemporary Britain old age has come to be seen as a problem for society, and the ever-increasing number of older people are seen in some quarters as a drain upon health care resources. Arber and Ginn begin Chapter 8 by challenging the idea that the elderly are a burden on society, arguing that this view owes more to the ageism which is inherent in modern societies than it does to empirical evidence. They go on to demonstrate that the experience of health and illness in later life has to be understood in terms of the context of gender, social class and social policy. They conclude by warning of the dangers of rationing health care according to age and argue that sociological researchers can help to give a voice to older people.

The final section of the book looks at the social context of health care in contemporary Britain. In the 1990s there have been major, and contentious, reforms of health policy and a restructuring of the NHS. In his chapter on the politics of health care reform (Chapter 9) Baggott begins by looking at the presumed breakdown of the post-war consensus on health policy. He argues that a focus on party-political rhetoric obstructs our understanding of policy making in this field. Despite the ideas of the 'new right' which shaped the reforms of the 1990s, policy making in the Health service was also driven by pragmatic considerations. He concludes that the policy changes to the health service represent not a total breakdown of the post-war consensus, but a moving consensus reflecting changing economic and political circumstances.

Health professionals play a pivotal role in contemporary health care services. Drawing on a long-standing sociological interest in professionalisation and professionalism as part of the process of modernisation, Saks (Chapter 10) focuses on professionalism in health care. He examines some of the theoretical debates about the role of the professions and the meaning of professionalism in the context of the rise of the medical profession. He then considers whether or not medical dominance in health care is being eroded by the increasing professionalism of occupations allied to medicine including alternative medicine. The chapter concludes with an examination of some of the benefits and drawbacks of professionalism in health care.

During the course of the twentieth century the modernisation of British society has been accompanied by the transformation of patterns of death and the 'medicalisation' of experiences of dying. In Chapter 11 Field looks at the ways in which these have been shaped by demographic and structural changes in British society. In particular, he examines changing patterns of communication between health workers and those who are dying and the move from 'closed' towards 'open' awareness contexts in caring for dying people. Most of the sociological (and other) research about the care of dying people has focused upon those dying from cancer and modern hospice and palliative care services are largely restricted to such patients. Field therefore concludes the chapter by identifying some of the impediments to the attempts to extend palliative care services to those dying from long-term chronic conditions.

Most of the care of people who are ill takes place in their own homes and is provided by their partners and families. Chapter 12 by Veronica James reflects sociology's traditional concern with the relationship between the individual and society drawing upon some of the issues addressed in earlier chapters. James links the provision of 'unwaged care' by families and other 'lay' carers to the wider social constraints in contemporary society. She begins by examining the difficulties of establishing the extent and scope of such care and the policy implications which various definitions and classifications of carers have. She also considers the impact of long-term care in the home for those unpaid carers providing it. The chapter ends by examining the relationship of unwaged care to the statutory, commercial and voluntary sectors of health care which is characteristic of contemporary Britain, highlighting the individual and societal implications of the greater emphasis upon individual and family responsibility for care and the lessening of collective state responsibilities.

The book is designed to be read either cumulatively or on a chapter by chapter basis. Each chapter stands on its own but collectively the chapters provide a good view of the range of empirical work and conceptual issues which currently exercise those working in the sociology of health and illness in Britain. The chapters focus both on issues of contemporary practical concern and demonstrate how sociology can be used to inform knowledge and understanding of these. Although the substantive focus is contemporary British society, the conceptual and methodological issues discussed have a wider contemporary relevance for sociologists in Europe, North America and elsewhere.

References

Bond, J. & Bond, S. (1994) *Sociology and Health Care: An Introduction for Nurses and Other Health Professions*, (2nd edn.) Churchill Livingstone, Edinburgh.

Bury, M. (1997) *Health and Illness in a Changing Society*. Routledge, London.

Freidson, E. (1988) *Profession of Medicine: A Study of the Sociology of Applied Knowledge*. University of Chicago, Chicago.

Gerhardt, U. (1989) *Ideas about Illness: An Intellectual and Political History of Medical Sociology*. Macmillan, London.

Nettleton, S. (1996) *The Sociology of Health and Illness*. Cambridge University Press, Cambridge.

Scambler, G. (ed) (1987) *Sociological Theory and Medical Sociology*. Tavistock, London.

Scambler, G. (ed) (1994) *Sociology as Applied to Medicine*, 4th edn. Ballière Tindall, London.

Taylor, S. & Field, D. (1997) *Sociology of Health and Health Care*, 2nd edn. Blackwell Science, Oxford.

Townsend, P. Davidson, N. & Whitehead, M. (1988) *Inequalities in Health: The Black Report/The Health Divide*. Penguin, Harmondsworth.

Turner, B. (1995) *Medical Power and Social Knowledge*, 2nd edn. Sage, London.

Part I
Conceptualisation and Research

Chapter 1
Conceptualising Chronic Illness

Michael P. Kelly and David Field

Introduction

This chapter links the sociological analysis of chronic illness with recent debates about changing social structures in contemporary Western society suggesting that, in view of the rapidly changing nature of that society, sociological conceptualisations of chronic illness need some reconsideration. Our argument is that two separate, but related, phenomena require us to reconsider the way that chronic illness has been conceptualised in medical sociology. The phenomena in question are: first, the way that advanced industrial societies are changing (sometimes called the transition to post-modernity) and, second, the body of theoretical ideas that have been developed to describe those changes (sometimes called post-modernism). It is not our purpose to enter into the debates about the precise sociocultural configuration of contemporary society, nor to assess the finer points of the theories. However, the various debates about post-modernity and post-modernism serve to highlight the Euro-centric and historically specific nature of the concepts which have dominated the sociology of chronic illness. It will be argued that the changing social structures of post-modern societies, and the theories about them, suggest that the theoretical precepts that have dominated sociological accounts of chronic illness need re-evaluation. This is not because these precepts were wrong. Rather, they were shaped by, and based upon, a particular view of the industrial societies in which they were formulated.

Initial sociological conceptualisations

The signal contribution of sociology to the understanding of chronic illness was its holistic approach to a variety of different chronic diseases.

This emphasis on the common social aspects of chronic illness is a feature of all the main medical sociological paradigms dealing with chronic illness. We distinguish two such paradigms: the socio-structural and the interactionist. Those writers focusing on the socio-structural we further sub-divide into structural-functionalists (and those influenced by structural-functionalism) and political economists.

The socio-structural conceptualisations focus deterministically on the impact of the illness on the individual, their family, work and leisure. The basic assumption underlying the structural-functionalist approach is that being chronically ill is a biological circumstance which forces an individual to live differently from their customary mode. This is because chronic disease results in a state of economic, social and psychological being that is discontinuous from the normal (Dingwall 1976: 62). The structural-functionalist approach, and those influenced by it, described how the biological pathology of chronic disease expanded beyond the individual sufferer's body, to a network of social relationships and interrupted their functioning. Chronic illness is thus conceptualized as a 'fault-line' across social attachments (Moos & Tsu 1977).

While not always working in an explicit structural-functional perspective, these ideas have helped to illuminate a range of difficulties and problems (Albrecht 1976). The key writer though, is Parsons (1951). He defined elements of behaviour and social relationships and, in the face of illness, the ways they would be disturbed, and then equilibrium re-established. In the Parsonian view of sickness, normal social functioning is interrupted, ordinary role responsibilities are relinquished, special relationships with the medical profession are established, and negative moral evaluations are _not_ applied to this state of affairs by the world at large. All of this, for Parsons, is defined within a normative framework in which illness is negatively perceived. Parsons' concepts were developed to describe acute illness, but the kinds of disturbances in the various systems and sub-systems of social and emotional networks, which were the concern of structural functionalism, can be, and have been applied to chronic illness quite helpfully (Moos & Tsu 1977).

The second socio-structural approach – political economy – although distinct from structural-functionalism, shares its deterministic orientation. Attention is focused this time, however, upon the ways in which chronic illness is produced by the capitalist system and the ways in which the distribution and management of chronic illness is related to Western industrial economies (e.g. Navarro 1976). The determinism operates from a socio-economic rather than a biological basis. Thus the production of commodities affects health both directly (e.g. through occupationally caused diseases and industrial pollution) and indirectly (e.g. by the marketing of tobacco products). As with the ownership of other commodities, health and illness are differentially distributed along social class lines, with lower social classes experiencing higher levels of illness and disability than higher social classes.

Political-economy sometimes also suggests that doctors and other 'health professionals' are agents of the state since medicine functions as an institution of social control. Further, the health care services are a part of the profit-based capitalist system, so 'health decisions' such as the adoption of a new drug or item of medical technology, are shaped by considerations of profit. Not only does the organisation of capitalist society have these detrimental consequences for the health and well-being of its population, but also the industrial world creates and exports ill health to developing countries by setting up unhealthy factories, exporting health damaging products and promoting unhealthy practices such as the use of substitutes for breast milk (Doyal 1981).

The two socio-structural approaches are the sociological analogues of the pathogenic approach of medical science identified by Antonovsky (1981). They are both thoroughly modernist in their assumptions about causation, and rely on the idea of 'system' to explicate the relationships upon which they focus. Antonovsky argued that most natural and social scientific disciplines have as their dominant approach, a systemic view of their subject matter. These systems may be biological, physical, sub-atomic, social or economic. However, he argued that systems-type thinking and a consideration of the characteristics of the systems, are dominant epistemological characteristics of most science. The principal analytic focus for the scientist is understanding system breakdown. The term Antonovsky used to describe the search for the causes of system breakdown was pathogenesis. In the structural-functional and the political economy approaches to chronic illness, the systemic breakdown is not bodily malfunction *per se*, but social malfunction or deviance. The difference is that for the structural-functionalists the bodily malfunction is the causal variable, whereas for the political economists, it is the outcome. Either way, both rest on a systems approach, and both are pathogenic in orientation. Both are products of a type of sociology grounded in a view of society as a relatively stable system – and the people within it as products of that system.

Antonovsky's insight was not only to alert us to the similarities between disciplines in their pathogenic approach, but also to suggest an alternative. The opposite of pathogenesis was, he argued, salutogenesis. Antonovsky meant by salutogenesis, the origins of health. The concern in salutogenesis is how people survive in a hostile world, and why systems persist and endure, rather than exploration of the origins of system failure or of ill health. It poses the question of how is it that so many people survive relatively intact given that the world so is full of hazards and risks, and that stressors of a microbiological, psychological, social, political, economic and physical kind are ubiquitous. The origins of health, he suggests, are to be found in the resources which facilitate this survival. Although not articulated in this way, the other sociological paradigm we describe below, the interactionist approach, actually deals with survival and adaptation, and most importantly does not assume a priori and inevitably that chronic illness is only a negative experience.

Interactionism goes much further than a description of disruption therefore, and is concerned with the meaning of illness and the construction, negotiation and transmission of that meaning. Thus methodologies which use qualitative techniques to allow sufferers to articulate in their own words the feelings of being ill, have been prominent (Strauss *et al.* 1984). Similarly, the use of concepts from parallel subspecialities within interactionism such as 'career', taken from the sociology of occupations, has been a feature of this type of literature. There is a large body of writing in this tradition, American and British, which shares a mission to 'tell it how it is' and to bring human suffering to the forefront of the analysis in a way in which the authors who concentrate on social systems and on disrupted normative frameworks, do not (e.g. Roth & Conrad 1987, Strauss *et al.* 1984).

The interactionist approach may itself be subdivided into two types of emphasis, one concentrating on crisis as a process, the other on self as a process (Gerhardt 1989). Early work, in particular, tended to focus on the crisis created by chronic illness or major disability. For example, Davis' classic study of childhood polio is titled *Passage through Crisis* (Davis 1963). In it he describes the ways in which families grapple with the uncertainties which characterise the recognition of apparently normal symptoms as actually constituting polio, and how they come to recognise and interpret the seriousness of their child's condition, and then struggle with the further uncertainties surrounding the nature and extent of the child's recovery. Davis' analysis of the breakdown of 'normalisation', the interpretation of social, physical and environmental cues, and the medical uses of uncertainty in the management of meaning in the social construction of the 'illness career', provided a model for many subsequent studies of chronic illness. Other examples of this genre are studies of blindness (Scott 1969) and of parents of children with disabilities (Voysey 1975). The emphasis is upon the fundamental alteration of the meaning of social life and of personal identities and their often difficult reconstitution following the usually sudden and unexpected appearance of the condition. Unlike the socio-structural approaches, which assume that illness undermines the social world, and that this by definition is invariably a negative experience, the interactionists attend to the way meaning is constructed and reconstructed by the participants in the social experiences of illness, and examine the ways in which negative and positive constructions of meaning are generated, sustained and changed.

In later work in interactionism the emphasis shifted to the analysis of more gradual transformations of self, identity and the social experiences which result from the physical and social deterioration of long-term chronic illness (Strauss *et al.* 1984). The epicentre of the analysis is the way self does (or does not) maintain a sense of continuity in the face of the identity changes which are the accompaniment to the (downward) status transition (Charmaz 1983). For these writers, the longevity of the experience, the extent to which changes in meaning are substantial and permanent or transient and fleeting, the degrees to which a discourse or accounting process can aid coping and the consequent transformation of self are explored (Kelly 1992). In theoretical terms, the attention is directed to the conflicts between self and public constructions of identity or labels. The sufferers' sense of being in the world and their disengagement from and re-engagement with others' perceptions, attitudes and behaviours towards them, constitute a fulcrum of analysis which allows the central life dilemmas of the chronically ill person to be described.

Each of the broad sociological approaches we have briefly reviewed above focus upon different aspects of chronic illness and draw upon different analytic frameworks and concepts in their analyses. Notwithstanding these theoretical differences and the strongly qualitative and sometimes phenomenological approach of the interactionists compared to the more formal preoccupations of the social-structuralists, it is the similarities between the approaches which are of most interest for the purposes of the rest of this chapter. The particular view of the nature of society shared by 'structural' and 'interpretative' writers is of a society which is ordered and stable and in which chronic illness breaks up or threatens that order at particular analytic levels. The social and economic worlds (namely modern Western industrial society dominated by manufacturing industry) are assumed to be relatively enduring and constant, and provide a fixed backdrop. Whether that backdrop is conceptualised as a system or as a negotiated reality does not matter. It is the continuity and predictability of the social world that is assumed and that is the basis on which the analysis proceeds. While some writers like Navarro (1976) may well define illness as a product of capitalism and see capitalism as undesirable in itself, they share with all writers of a modernist persuasion an ontology in which social order is paramount. The analyses of authors like Parsons (1951) and Bury (1982) (to take two very different approaches) shift the emphasis to the processes of adaptation following the disruption, nevertheless their background assumptions are of an orderly, enduring and predictable social world in which illness is a social or symbolic pathogen.

The similarity of the approaches in large part flows from their shared ethnocentric model of society: Western advanced industrial (capitalist) society. The notion of illness as disruption assumes *a priori* a sufficient stability to be disrupted and a Cartesian notion of self to be objectified. The social world is seen as one in which the division of labour is complex and refined, but well understood by the society's members. Within that division of labour are well known anchor points of social structure and individual meaning, such as age, gender, class, politics and work. These familiar, well-understood aspects of everyday life form the basis for the taken for granted structure of people's lives and also the taken for granted foci of sociological analysis. For example, in the literature divisions of gender and ethnicity in the experience of chronic illness were scarcely commented upon and even the discussion of social class divisions were frequently reduced to little more than the a-theoretical discussion of occupational classification.

Our point is that the forms of sociological analysis of chronic illness described above are locked into a very particular socio-historical time – modernity – and a very particular social analysis of that time – modernism – and that the understanding of chronic illness in other types of society e.g. pre-modern, contemporary non-western, or even post-modern societies, may require different analytic constructs. Anthropology and cross-cultural studies fill the gap to some extent, although it is worth noting that their impact on mainstream British medical sociological studies of chronic illness has not been great. Of more interest to us is the appropriateness of these types of analysis as we move into a social world in which many of the certainties of late modern society disappear or become distorted. The sociological approaches of the socio-structuralists and interactionists described above, may no longer be wholly appropriate even to those societies of North America and Western Europe, which generated them. At the very least, the postmodern turn in sociology should force us to rethink some of the assumptions of this type of analysis.

Some trends in late modernity

Many commentators have noted that in advanced industrial societies, the nature of social and economic life has changed in a number of significant ways (Lyotard 1984). Others have suggested that the nature of social theory itself must fundamentally change in order to capture the nature of a changing social reality (Bauman 1992). Our argument is that the social changes to the contemporary societies have had a potentially profound effect on the nature of the experience of chronic illness. We also consider whether some of the theoretical ideas which have been used to describe these changes – post modernism – may take the analysis of chronic illness forward.

It has been argued that post-modernity (the world which post-modernism describes) is a world in which aesthetics supersedes practicalities. It is a world in which conventional social arrangements are said to be deconstructed and in which experimentation in cultural, artistic and lifeforms predominate. (Lyotard 1984, Bauman 1992). The core idea of post-modernity is that the social and moral conditions of the present mark a fundamental break with the past. In art, form displaces content; in philosophy, interpretation displaces system; in politics, pragmatism displaces principle; in science chaos displaces order. Post-modernity therefore refers to a major social, and cultural disjunction that is alleged to have happened in various fields of human and scientific endeavour, and indeed to society itself, especially in the twentieth century. This has been particularly associated with the discrediting and questioning of the possibility of ultimate truth and/or human happiness being revealed or produced by science.

For all of this to make sense, an idea of what post-modernity is about, is helpful. Modernity had originally been defined with reference to its difference from the traditional order which preceded it. Modernity and the theories which described it (including most sociological theory) implied a progressive economic and administrative rationalisation and differentiation of the social world (Crook *et al.* 1992) which was an advance on traditional society. Post-modernity suggests an epochal shift or break with this and the sense of progress it implied. Post-modernity involves, so the argument goes, the emergence of a new social order in which instead of progress there is only change. Modernity was based on a fundamental belief that there was an absolute bedrock of rational truth which scientific enquiry was working to reveal. The post-modern view is that ultimate truth does not exist. Modernity was the attempt to impose structures on a disorderly traditional world (Bauman 1992). Post-modernity is the celebration of disorderliness and the recognition of the impossibility of anything other than imperfect and temporary structures of meaning to help understand the disorderly world.

We do not subscribe to this post-modern view in full, in any sense. We suggest, in contrast, that the contemporary social world in Western Europe and North America consists of a number of continuities and discontinuities with the past. Post-modernism throws some light on these discontinuities in particular. What we want to show is how the interplay between these continuities and discontinuities, affects the experience of chronic illness. Thus, what we attempt here is to identify those key social changes in contemporary Western European and North American societies which have resulted in the refashioning of social institutions and organisations, the appearance of new forms of social configuration and new types of social conduct which have had consequences for the experience of chronic illness.

We look first at the economic base and the work roles arising in the economic base which original sociological conceptualisations of chronic illness (either implicitly or explicitly) placed as central to understanding the disruption of social life. Industrial societies defined work roles and careers as relatively fixed and lifelong (and indeed interactionists used the idea of career to describe illness itself as a substitute status for work!). This, we suggest, has been overtaken – many work roles have been fundamentally altered. The transition from a manufacturing-based economy to a predominantly service economy and contingent developments in information technology, automation and the introduction of more flexible working patterns, have led to the widespread disappearance of industrial work dependent upon predominantly male, low skilled manual labour. Traditional jobs linked to primary production and to manufacturing have disappeared by the million. New types of segmented labour markets have emerged in which part-time and short-term work in retail, leisure and service sectors predominate. The number of women in employment, mainly in these areas, has increased significantly. The growth of global markets, and consumerism are important economic developments which have been accompanied by diminishing state intervention into economic and social aspects of life. Governments do not appear to find it politically necessary, desirable or perhaps possible to try to run full employment economies, for example.

Against this economic background, the important social divisions of class, age, gender and party politics which were arguably once fundamental and accepted axes of social structure and identity have become more fluid and less deterministic. In Britain, for example, local and national party politics appear to have become far less class based than they once were and voting patterns reflect the loosening of class allegiances and voluntary disenfranchisement. Gender identities have become less rigid and coercive and cultural identities based upon ethnicity are more prominent, highlighting a range of legitimate diversity not previously acknowledged. As these axes of differentiation in society cease to hold such sway, new ones emerge to vie for practical and analytic attention. Fashion and image, particularly among the young, have become more important in a world greatly touched by mass media and rapid mass communication where there are no absolute standards or 'ultimate truths'. There appears to be a lack of authoritative social institutions to give meaning, shape and coherence to social life. For example, in Britain social institutions such as the police, the National Health Service, the school and university systems have been destabilised as the consequence of deregulation and the operation of market forces. Others, like the monarchy and the Christian churches, appear to have abandoned their earlier roles as sources of normative and legitimate authority. The sorts of domestic lives people lead also reflects this range of diversity and fragmentation. While marriage continues to be popular, divorce rates are high and single parenthood, serial monogamy, multi-children families in non-consanguineous cohabitation, same sex partnerships and single households have all come to be defined as available and legitimate alternatives.

It would, of course, be quite naive to say that families no longer exist, or that no one ever votes along class lines, or believes in God, or works their way through a traditional career in a branch of manufacturing industry. Neither would it make any kind of sociological or historical sense to suggest that 30, 60, or 90 years ago there was a fixed and unchanging social world in which the social structure was stable and which was a much better place to live in. However, the pace of social change has altered. The increasingly rapid fragmentation of institutions and reshaping of social forms poses some very serious questions about the nature of contemporary society and certain aspects of it, including chronic illness.

The experience of chronic illness in contemporary British society

Our aim in this section is to suggest how contemporary experiences of chronic illness need to be understood in terms of the changing contexts of western society. We suggest that not only have the social structures of contemporary western societies become more diffuse and fragmented but the experiences of chronic illness have also become more diverse. In 'high modernity' the classic Parsonian 'sick role' defined the experience of illness adequately (as occupational and family roles did for the broader social structure and life experience). In a world of more fragmented social structures a new conceptualisation of the variety of the experience of chronic illnesses is required.

The changes to social organisation and social structure just described, impact on the lifeworld, and it is here we begin our analysis. Schutz (1970) defined the lifeworld as the everyday taken for granted aspects of the familiar, routine and immediate experience of ordinary men and women. The lifeworld consists of the relationships and mundane realities through which, and in which, people make sense of the world that is known to them. It also provides the means to understand the world they know exists beyond their immediate experience.

For Schutz, the lifeworld was grounded in a notion of experience which was circumscribed physically and temporally. The social world that humans inhabit is foreclosed and in part limited by the functional capacity of the body. In a very materialist sense, the capacity to move, walk, and interact and the physical distance that a body can manoeuvre within a given time period, to a large degree determines the parameters of interactional possibilities and the nature of the here and now of experience. The number of people and places that the human can know well, or indeed can even be familiar with, is finite. The circumscribed world of everyday life is one of familiar people and things – like one's own body. It is the world of everyday routines and mundane experiences, including bodily functions. It is a world of social experience that is taken for granted. Such is its familiarity and its known qualities, that it contains few surprises and even fewer reasons to engage in self-reflexivity. The body is a component of this taken for granted reality which goes by largely unnoticed until such times as illness or other things impinge on it, causing time for reflection and a reconsideration of the meanings of the familiar things around and in the person (Kelly 1992, Kelly & Field 1996).

According to Schutz, beyond the worlds of immediate experience there are worlds that are not especially familiar, but which the person knows exists and which they might reasonably expect to have contact with at some point in their lives. These include ideas about what it might be like to be old, ill, or disabled, as well as what it might be like to be somewhere far away. Still further away from the worlds of immediate and anticipated experience are lives and environments which, while known, exist in the mind as little more than a theoretical possibility rather than anything very concrete.

The immediate and potential lifeworlds of individuals are private and yet shared with others. They are private because the understandings and sensations and perceptions which exist in the minds of the individual, of self, are not directly knowable to others other than in the ways that an individual chooses to reveal them to others, usually in talk, although this may also be achieved by the appearance and bodily presentation of self and identity (Goffman 1959). In most interactions, however, people make the routine assumption that the world is experienced and perceived in much the same way by others, as by self, and that broadly what is going on around the individual, has the same approximate meanings to others also. This Schutz called intersubjectivity.

Schutz was writing before television, video recorders, mobile telephones and the Internet had been invented. He was also writing against the fixed anchor points of social differentiation based on a stable economic (industrial) base. With their advent, mass media communications and also 'do it yourself' communications have shifted and expanded the boundaries of the lifeworld by creating a new type of experience, expanding the potentially knowable, and giving a new basis for inter-subjectivity. The 'face to faceness' of relationships has been expanded and also changed as a consequence of modes of communications which allow direct immediate interaction at a distance. This has played a part in the general fragmentation of social life. One consequence of the evolution of 'do it yourself' communications on a mass scale seems to have been the 'privatisation' of communications in the sense of a social and domestic world turning in on itself. Such communications are qualitatively different from the reception of mass communications whose content and form is controlled editorially by States or capitalist organisations.

Using the Internet, for example, is a very different type of experience from physical face to face interaction and is symptomatic of other cultural processes involving both the expansion of individual choice and control and the privatisation of the lifeworld. In respect of chronic illness, the multiple and unregulated avenues of communication provide the potential for greater communication between those with chronic illness, potentially expanding the range of explanations and understandings of chronic conditions, many of them contrary to, or critical of, dominant medical definitions. In this sense it could perform important informational and support functions. It could also legitimatise the experiences of sufferers by putting them in touch with others in a similar position. There are also clear political uses which are possible, such as mobilising support for or against local and national policy initiatives. Thus, there are potentially empowering aspects for people with chronic illness as the Internet facilitates their capacity to make choices independently of 'official' (medicalised) definitions, resources and policy structures.

In interactionist accounts, chronic illness has conventionally been treated as a dominant and all-pervasive identity. We define identity as the public knowable and known aspect of the person in which social structure, in the form of social roles, interacts with person (Kelly 1992). In modern industrial societies, the societies in which the medical sociology of chronic illness evolved, identities were varied and linked to the division of labour. However, for any given individual the number of identities which they might assume was circumscribed. This was because the anchor points of social roles were themselves relatively limited to the core identities of occupation, community, gender, age and religion. These identities had an enduring quality through time. Geographical and social mobility were finite, and short distance for most people, and the identities were frequently life-long. Post-war British sociology is replete with studies that demonstrate precisely these features of social life, especially for the working class life (e.g. Ashton & Field 1976).

In a very important sense, the identity of being chronically ill in such social structures mirrored the core identities in the social structure. To be chronically sick was to occupy a particular identity (an alternative career) over a long period of time. Being chronically ill was for many a dominant status and, very importantly, the chronically ill identity displaced the 'normal' identities of work, leisure and family life in the disruptive way the literature discussed above described. The identity of the chronically sick person was defined almost exclusively with reference to a medical definition of the situation and the medical profession were the arbiters of the role through their diagnostic criteria and their legitimising role in accessing clinical, social and financial services. Much of this still holds true, particularly among the less affluent. However, in contemporary North American and Western European societies, the nature of identity has become a great deal more fragmented, as the core identities of work, family and leisure have been reshaped by the social changes we have already described.

According to Giddens (1991), in this fluid and open social world individuals are forced to become self-reflexive and to construct their own life styles rather than being able to accept pre-given, socially scripted roles and identities as guides to their behaviour. This is not to say that there are no role models or guides, for individual life styles can be constructed by drawing upon the wide range of options which are available in the highly commodified, media saturated 'post-modern' world. Managing and presenting the right appearance may become central to (and indeed may become the totality of) the maintenance of such identities and life styles. The implications of this for chronic illness, as we shall develop further, are that the chronic illness identities may be less coercive and constraining in post-modern than in modern times.

We have noted the importance of appearance for identity. The literature inspired by Goffman (1963) made the issue of appearance, and especially spoiled appearance, central to its analysis and linked it to both public identity and self conception. Whatever other sophistications and nuances subsequent authors added, the inescapable premise, the debt to Goffman, was that appearance may be constructed in such a way as to be negatively evaluated by self and by others and that this negatively defined difference constituted the central problem for the person and others with whom they interacted. This assumption used to pervade the literature on chronic illness. However, more recently there appears to have been a change in the discourse about the appearance of those who are chronically ill and/or have a disability. Inspired by post-modernism in general and the disability movement in particular, there is not only a celebration of difference, but also an explicit attack on what is defined as the ideological assumption that difference is bad (Shakespeare, 1996). This leads not only to a kind of relativism in the aesthetics of appearance but also to a demand for tolerance of difference. The discourse of difference has produced a parallel universe of discourse to the world of the non-ill, or non-disabled, in which issues pertaining to chronic illness and to disability may be articulated, out of the gaze of the world at large, and in a way that identities independent of the illness or the disability can be sustained and developed.

So far we have concentrated on the 'public' aspect of identity. We now turn to consider the private, subjective, aspect of the self which we see as structured in narrative and in talk with others (Kelly & Dickinson 1997). Mead (1934) argued that the crucial human capacity to objectify the self was facilitated by linguistic forms and located in discourse. Informing his analysis is the view that such discourse drew upon (and established for the individual) an external (social) world which could be taken for granted as an orderly and continuous place. Outside the academic world, the self of the modern era was typically talked about in a taken for granted way and was seldom the object of detailed analysis other than in certain types of literary forms like the novel. In the post-modern world where external certainties have ceased to have quite the same degree of concreteness and coherence, self may be perceived by many more people as fragmented and lacking a strong centre taking on a kind of hyper-reflexivity and intensive monitoring which fits a world of uncertainty. In certain sectors of society, under the influence of psychoanalysis, or other hyper-discourses of self, the self has not only become an object of analysis, but an industry in its own right.

We suggest that the discourses which people can draw upon to talk about themselves have thus changed and that this in turn potentially affects the narratives of chronic illness. The issues for chronic illness sufferers are twofold. First, we have noted that in modern societies chronic illness was seen as creating uncertainty in a world of relative certainty. Much of the social scientific description of chronic illness which has dominated medical sociology has been precisely about the search for certainty (for system or meaning) in the face of an unpredictable illness. In the contemporary world, in which chronic illness is just one more uncertainty in a continually changing and uncertain world, then the discourse of sufferers will be about coping with chronic illness. The social scientific discourses, are also going to be about coping in a world in which illness is just another problem or burden; just one among many stressors or assaults that the individual has to contend with. The psychology of coping given in the later work of Lazarus (Lazarus & Folkman 1984), and the salutogenic paradigm of Antonovsky (1981) (above) provide the social scientific touchstone to that new discourse. For both Lazarus and Antonovsky the acknowledgement is made quite explicitly that human life is one of difficulty and travail. The human condition is characterised as endemically stressful and problematic.

A second important change which has implications for the identity and self of chronically ill people is the increasing challenge to the hegemony of medicine. Whereas the medical profession once had *carte blanche* to define the sick role in chronic disease, now a whole range of others seek to do so, and have acquired a legitimacy so to do. These include alternative medicine, a mass media for whom illness, including chronic illness, is a form of entertainment, and disease specific local and national 'self help' organisations. It is relatively easy to learn about these pluralistic responses to illness, because each has its own narrative form in popular culture. We can learn 'how to cope' in the pages of a magazine, we can watch chronic illness being normalised in the tri-weekly soap opera, and all manner of mass media will tell us about the wonders of modern medical science and the alternative advantages of 'holistic' treatment regimes.

These discourses about chronic illness are linked to a range of issues relating to politics, liberation, victimology, coping, self-help, counselling, finding one's true self and so on. For example, for the Disability Alliance chronic illness is a form of political consciousness and action and the explanation of illness and disability are as much to do with ideology and counter-ideology, as anything else. In other words there are a variety of ways of potentially 'doing' chronic illness and of being ill, which reach well beyond the conventional boundaries of medicine and into a number of different fields of human activity. In the modern era, when the medical hegemony was a great deal more absolute than it is now, the medical profession was able to dominate the definition and management of chronic illness. Presently, medical discourse, while still significant is certainly not the only explanation which sick people can draw upon to try to find a way of understanding their self and identity within the world. The competing definitions of the disability movement, the panoply of alternative medicine, as well as the 'old fashioned' lay and religious beliefs about illness, and many others provide a set of parallel discourses between which little meaningful communication takes place.

Another relevant concept is that of time. In early modern industrial societies individual time-lines could be described as relatively short, but continuous and relatively differentiated. Chronic disease cut the timeline. It not only caused discontinuity in the line itself, but probably made it shorter as well. In contemporary Western Europe and North America, individual time-lines are longer but much less well defined. Life itself has lost some of its certainties and continuities by virtue of the economic, technological and social changes described above. If life itself is discontinuous, then the disruptive consequences of chronic illness may be less marked. In this respect chronic illness is one among a number of potential causes of changing life styles. Although for some individuals it may cause as much disruption and disorder as in modern society, it may provide a focus for stability, continuity and identity for other individuals whose lives were already disjoined in various ways.

So far we have concentrated upon the consequences of changing patterns of social life for the experience of chronic illness. We therefore conclude this section by briefly considering the 'material basis' of chronic illness: the body that is diseased. Here the impact of medical technology is important. More effective drug management regimes and new types of surgery have had profoundly liberating effects for some types of chronic disease allowing the possibility of living life at 'arm's length' from the illness and thus from a life completely swamped by the condition. That is, the extent of discontinuity and disruption is potentially contained and minimised. This, in turn, allows people to maintain other identities in work and domestic life. In these circumstances chronic illness, although remaining an important basis for identity, does not become *the* dominant identity. Ironically, the control of disease through medicine facilitates and undermines medicine itself. It allows the sufferer to live more independently of medicine than might once have been the case and potentially delegitimises medicine's role in defining the situation.

Reconceptualising the experience of chronic illness

We began this chapter by identifying a number of commonalities in sociological approaches to chronic illness: the stress on the similarities across the range of chronic illnesses, the difference of chronic illness from 'normal life', the focus on its disruptive consequences, and the emphasis upon the importance of social contexts. Although the emphasis upon the similarities of experiences across the range of chronic illnesses is important, there does seem to be a case for serious consideration of the range of experiences of chronic illness. More recent work has indeed begun to analyse not only the 'sameness in difference' but also the differences between conditions and, equally important, the differences between individuals in the experiences of the same or similar conditions.

We have argued that there is a greater range of discourses to make

sense of chronic illness, and that the dominance of the medical hegemony is breaking down. This needs to be examined in more detail, and
with reference to particular conditions. We have also argued that the
bases for identity and self conception are more fluid and less coercive
than previously, but the implications of this for the impact of chronic
illness on personal life have been scarcely addressed. As we have suggested, there are now potentially a number of different options available
for 'doing' chronic illness.

The analytic stress on differences between different experiences of
chronic illness and styles of 'doing' or coping with it should not, however, retain the assumption so deeply embedded in earlier sociological
conceptualisations that having a chronic illness excludes individuals
from normal life. To some extent this assumption was undercut by the
emphasis in many sociological writings on the 'normalisation' of life by
chronically ill people and their families. While in this literature it is clear
that people came to terms in various ways with 'living with their condition' and that for many of them once this had happened they were able
to lead lives which were not substantially different in most respects from
other people, this was not given due analytic weight. By focusing upon
disruption and difference, e.g. describing how people 'reconstructed
good and evil' or 'discovered true values' (Voysey 1975), their work
towards a positive acceptance of their altered being was somehow
reduced to a 'trick' of 'normalisation'. Their normality was ersatz and
fundamentally different from 'proper' normality. That is, the analysis
served to remind the reader that such individuals and families were not
really normal. With the greater apparent diversity of contemporary
lifestyles it is increasingly hard to maintain that position with any con-
viction. Further, as chronic illness is so much a part of everyday life (in
1994 nearly one-fifth of the respondents to the General Household
Survey reported their activities were restricted by a long-standing illness
(OPCS 1996)), it is hard to argue that it is not normal.

It may also be that chronic illness is not necessarily disruptive. For
some people at least it does not seem to be any more disruptive of life
than other common life changes. In part this reflects the changing, more
fragmented, social contexts of contemporary society life – and hence of
chronic illness – as much as it does more effective management of
chronic conditions. In particular, work and chronic illness are no longer
in a necessarily 'oppositional' relationship. Advances in the medical
treatment and management of chronic illness further weaken the disruptive impact of many conditions. Among the many bases available for
identity construction, chronic illness may become a stable orienting
aspect of individuals' lives, providing shape, meaning and coherence to
them and articulating social contact. Further, the narrow definition of

what is and is not normal has been replaced by the recognition (if not always acceptance) of a range of appearances and lifestyles. That is, 'normality' itself is seen as more differentiated and relativistic, encompassing an increasingly wider range of 'differences in normality'. Thus, the assumption that chronic illness will inevitably disrupt normal patterns of life in a pathological manner is no longer valid, or at least its validity is a theoretical problem.

Conclusions

We have highlighted a range of continuities and discontinuities in contemporary Western societies compared to their modern predecessors, in which the major paradigms of medical sociology developed. We suggest that the tensions between these continuities and discontinuities require that some of the standard sociological concepts used to describe and analyse chronic illness need reconsideration. On the one hand, contemporary societies offer a great range of explanatory discourses about chronic illness and the potential for greater and more effective control of certain bodily manifestations of chronic illness. There also seems to be greater tolerance – and even celebration – of diversity and difference within an expanded range of what is deemed to be normal. Thus, in a world of less determinative social structures, there is the potential for the experience of chronic illness to be less disruptive and 'non-normal' than in modern societies. On the other hand, the bodily limitations and activity restrictions caused by chronic illnesses cannot be completely ignored. Further, chronic illness is still linked to material deprivation and the experience of it is undoubtedly made more difficult in situations of deprivation; thus, for many people chronic illness is still greatly life limiting. While, as we have suggested, the old paradigms are now in need of revision or replacement, any new paradigm must be able to embrace both the change and diversity of post-modern society and the continuing physical and material bases of chronic illness.

References

Albrecht, G.L. (1976) Socialization and the disability process. In: *The Sociology of Disability and Rehabilitation* (ed. G.L. Albrecht). University of Pittsburg, Pittsburgh.

Antonovsky, A. (1981) *Health, Stress and Coping*. Jossey-Bass, San Francisco & London.

Ashton, D.N. & Field, D. (1976) *Young Workers: From School to Work*. Hutchinson, London.

Bauman, Z. (1992) *Intimations of Post-modernity*. Routledge, London.

Bury, M. (1982) Chronic illness as biographical disruption. *Sociology of Health and Illness*, **5**, 168–95.

Charmaz, C. (1983) Loss of self: a fundamental form of suffering in the chronically ill. *Sociology of Health and Illness*, **5**, 168–95.

Crook, S., Pakulski, J. & Waters, M. (1992) *Postmodernisation: Change in Advanced Society*. Sage, London.

Davis, F. (1963) *Passage through Crisis: Polio Victims and their Families*. Bobbs-Merrill, Indianapolis.

Dingwall, R. (1976) *Aspects of Illness*. Martin Robertson, London.

Doyal, L. (1981) *The Political Economy of Health*. Pluto Press, London.

Gerhardt, U. (1989) *Ideas about Illness: An Intellectual and Political History of Medical Sociology*. Macmillan, London.

Giddens, A. (1991) *Modernity and Self Identity: Self and Society in the Late Modern Age*. Polity, Oxford.

Goffman, E. (1959) *The Presentation of Self in Everyday Life*. Doubleday Anchor, New York.

Goffman, E. (1963) *Stigma: Notes on the Management of Spoiled Identity*. Prentice Hall, Englewood Cliffs, NJ.

Kelly, M.P. (1992) *Colitis*. Tavistock/Routledge, London.

Kelly, M.P. & Dickinson, H. (1997) The narrative self in autobiographical accounts of illness. *The Sociological Review*, **45**, 254–78.

Kelly, M. & Field, D. (1996) Medical sociology, chronic illness and the body. *Sociology of Health and Illness*, **18**, 241–57.

Lazarus, R. & Folkman, S. (1984) Coping and adaptation. In: *Handbook of Behavioral Medicine* (ed. W.D. Gentry). The Guild Press, New York.

Lyotard, J.F. (1984) *The Post-modern Condition: A Report on Knowledge* (trans G. Bennington & B. Massumi). Manchester University, Manchester.

Mead, G.H. (1934) *Mind, Self and Society*. University of Chicago, Chicago.

Moos, R.H. & Tsu, V.D. (eds) (1977) *Coping with Physical Illness*. Plenum, New York.

Navarro, V. (1976) *Medicine under Capitalism*. Prodist, New York.

OPCS (Office of Population and Surveys) (1996) *Living in Britain: Results from the 1994 General Household Survey*. HMSO, London.

Parsons, T. (1951) *The Social System*. The Free Press, Glencoe, Illinois.

Roth, J. & Conrad, P. (eds) (1987) *The Experience and Management of Chronic Illness*. JAI, London.

Schutz, A. (1970) *On Phenomenology and Social Relations*. University of Chicago Press, Chicago.

Scott, R. (1969) *The Making of Blind Men*. Russell Sage Foundation, New York.

Shakespeare, T. (1996) Disability, identity, difference. In: *Exploring the Divide: Illness and Disability* (eds C. Barnes & G. Mercer). The Disability Press, Leeds. pp. 94–113.

Strauss, A.L., Corbin, J., Fagerhaugh, S., Suczek, B. & Wiener, C. (1984) *Chronic Illness and the Quality of Life*, (2nd edn). C.V. Mosby, St Louis.

Voysey M. (1975) *A Constant Burden: The Reconstitution of Family Life*. Routledge Kegan Paul, London.

Chapter 2
The Identification of Cases in Psychiatry

Lindsay Prior

Introduction

This chapter is concerned with the relationship between subjects and cases in psychiatric epidemiology and routine psychiatric work. It seeks to illustrate a number of common problems associated with the identification of subjects as cases, and then moves on to consider how social scientific researchers and health workers attempt to resolve such difficulties. In that respect, the chapter centres on issues surrounding the construction and deconstruction of cases. However, a more important issue concerns the ways in which cases are commonly defined in relation to organisational needs rather than the personal needs of clients and subjects. In that vein the chapter ends with a consideration of two notorious case histories which serve to highlight what goes wrong when psychiatric workers lose sight of the 'person' in their search for treatable cases. The chapter opens with reference to some findings from a recent OPCS survey of psychiatric morbidity in the community.

Subjects as cases

In a study of adults (aged 16–64) living in private households in Great Britain during 1993, the OPCS estimated that some 14% of individuals exhibited the existence of 'significant neurotic psychopathology' (Meltzer *et al.* 1995: 13). In addition to this, the authors of the OPCS study also provided estimates of prevalence rates for six neurotic disorders, together with estimates for the prevalence of functional psychosis, alcohol and drug dependence. The rates (by gender) are reported in Table 2.1.

Table 2.1 Prevalence rates for six neurotic disorders, functional psychoses, drug and alcohol addiction.

Disorder	Female	Male
	Age 16–64	
Rates per 1000 in one week:		
Mixed anxiety and depressive disorder	99	54
Generalised anxiety disorder	34	28
Depressive episode	25	17
All phobias	14	7
Obsessive-compulsive disorder	15	9
Rates per 1000 in 12 months:		
Functional psychoses	4	4
Alcohol dependence	21	75
Drug dependence	15	29

Source: Meltzer, H., Gill, B., Petticrew, M. & Hinds, K. (1995) *The Prevalence of Psychiatric Morbidity among Adults Living in Private Households*. OPCS Surveys of Psychiatric Morbidity in Great Britain. Report. 1. HMSO, London.

Understandably, the results of the OPCS survey rested on the identification of cases – in this instance cases drawn from a population of some 10 000 persons. There was, however, nothing natural or self-evident about the recognition of those cases. Indeed, in examining almost any description of the social world, whether it be of psychiatric morbidity or not, we are invariably drawn to the conclusion that 'Cases matter; [yet] there is nothing innocent in how they are framed', (White 1992: 84).

In terms of both psychiatry and social science, of course, a 'case' is usually (though not exclusively) regarded both as:

● a human subject, and
● something else that is exemplified through recognisable features of that subject.

As far as the study and organisation of psychiatric morbidity is concerned, these two aspects of caseness are forever intermingled. For example in Brown and Harris' study of depression (1978), the cases are initially construed as both individual women and as episodes of diagnosed depressive disorder. While in the OPCS study, referenced above, cases are initially conceptualised as the 10 108 adults who co-operated in the private household survey and, later, the instances of psychiatric morbidity eventually identified in the study. Now, as with most kinds of social scientific research, these surveys are predicated on the assumption that the base materials of psychiatric practice and of social scientific investigation, in general, are somehow locked 'in' the subject. As a result, the primary tasks of the social scientific researcher are believed to involve the extraction of information from the subject by the use of questionnaires, interactive interviews, discussion groups, and the like. Indeed, the implication seems to be that research instruments and procedures can be routinely and easily used so as to unzip what are considered to be naturally occurring packages of data which lay deep in the secret recesses of the isolated subject. It is this implication, among others, that I wish to question here.

The use of what may be called person-oriented research instruments to identify cases, does more than merely serve to underline the ways in which we regard social scientific data as the property of isolated subjects. Indeed, there are at least two other implications of their use that deserve consideration. First, that the human conditions being researched are readily identifiable 'natural kinds' ready and waiting 'out there' in the social world to be picked up and analysed. That is to say, they imply that instruments are mere nets by means of which natural kinds may be captured and that the nets themselves have only a negligible impact on the research data. Secondly, they imply that the identification of cases is primarily a technical matter of finding reliable and valid instruments and that application of the technical instruments will suffice to discriminate between proper and improper cases of 'X'. Thus, to invoke the Brown and Harris study, the Present State Examination (PSE) was used in their 'community' sample of 458 females, first to identify and then to weed out current cases of clinical depression. While the OPCS study used, among other instruments, the Clinical Interview Schedule (CIS-R), (Lewis & Pelosi 1990) to assess the extent of psychopathology. In both examples, then, we see (a) a focus on the subject, (b) the use of specific instruments as nets for gathering what might be called naturally occurring cases, and (c) the implication that accurate identification of cases is primarily a matter of objective, technical expertise.

One of the main aims of this chapter will be to highlight and underline the ways in which the identification of cases involves more than simple matters of technical judgement and expertise *vis à vis* the autonomous human subject. Indeed, and especially once we move beyond the research agenda, it seems more likely that they involve detailed consideration of the practical professional interests, mutual social relations and organisational needs and operations which ordinarily surround the subject. The latter, of course, besides any symptoms, signs or qualities believed to be contained within the subject.

It will be argued that cases have always to be manufactured or constructed in accordance with organisational imperatives before they can be analysed either in terms of social science or in terms of professional practice. In the social scientific context, Ragin (1992) has referred to the process of construction as 'casing' and has outlined the ways in which cases are necessary but nevertheless manufactured products of basic research operations. While Walton has argued that 'cases come wrapped in theories' (Walton 1992:122), and can only be recognised as cases of something in terms of theories. In this chapter, however, I would prefer to tilt this last insight toward practice, and assert that cases are produced in and through social practices – sometimes research practices of social scientists, and at other times the day-to-day practices of psychiatrists, nurses, social workers and the like. In neither framework, however, can one argue that caseness resides solely 'within' the subject.

Caseness, then, is something imposed on subjects from outside according to practical interests. In the realm of social research such interests often have few, if any, immediate consequences for the lives of people being studied (unless we begin to think in terms of action research). In the field of professional action, however, the recognition and imposition of caseness can, as we shall see, have very serious implications for all concerned. For a case is more than simply an instance of an illness. 'It is a way of constructing a person'. (Barrett 1996: 13).

My claims will be reviewed and supported in the sections which follow. Throughout, however, my primary point of focus will be on the complex relationship that exists between individual subjects, and subjects as 'cases for research' or 'cases for practice'. In this light, and as we shall see, one subject can usually be considered as providing the raw materials for any number of diverse cases – depending on how that subject relates to the practical frames of work and organisational procedures in which they become embroiled. In a research context, for example, one (isolated) subject may present themselves as plausible candidates for any one of a number of different classification categories. So, in the realm of psychiatric morbidity, a subject may display psychiatric symptoms belonging to more than one diagnostic category. Consequently rules of hierarchy and precedence will have to be devised by the researcher in order to classify satisfactorily a given person as 'a case of Y' rather than, say, 'a case of X'. In a more practical work-based and professional context, the subject might form the occasion for attention from any one of a number of professional intervention agencies, or even any one team from a number of different teams within the same agency. A case for social work might thus evolve into a case for psychiatry, or a case for psychiatry might be summarily demoted to a case for the housing department. In any event, 'cases' are most likely to be negotiated in relation to a complex mesh of social processes and organisational interests. As we shall see, that process of construction and negotiation can sometimes lead to sad and fatal consequences.

Cases as products of technical operations: the construction and deconstruction of subjects as cases

The following exchange is a report on a conversation between staff nurses. The conversation concerned a hospital patient. It occurred at the switch-over between the morning and afternoon shifts when the nurses routinely reported on the patients in their care. Staff Nurse 1 (SN1) is puzzled about why one particular patient is in the ward given that he has not displayed any of the common symptoms associated with a psychotic illness.

> **SN1:** Does anyone know what's supposed to be wrong with G?
> [There was no immediate answer to this question and several of the other nurses exchange glances of bewilderment]
> **SN2:** Schizophrenia I suppose.
> **SN1:** Humph. (Pause). I've never seen any sign of it.
> **SN3:** Well, he's on chlorpromazine so he must be schizophrenic.

In psychiatry, as in other fields of medicine, a case traditionally designated a patient and an illness simultaneously. The illness, considered as a discrete entity, was usually characterised (described, classified and identified) in fields of thought and action (such as pathology, epidemiology, nosology) which existed independently of the singular patient. Within such a context the task of a clinician was, in part, believed to involve an assessment as to whether a given patient did or did not measure up appropriately to the template of disease or disorder which lay at hand.

In the routine life of the hospital ward nurses, psychiatrists and other professionals are constantly shifting their attention between patients and their illnesses. In the context of the hospital above (Prior 1993), it was often difficult to separate the two, though distinctions were routinely made. This was especially so when patients showed evidence of being violent – whereupon the distinction between 'badness' and 'madness' was called upon to explain and justify the social relations which then held between a violent patient and the professionals. However, and as far as illness was concerned, psychiatrists and nurses tended to support what might be called the ontological theory of disease. That is to say, they believed that any given patient either 'had' or did not have such a disease or disorder. In my opening sequence, for example, the question was directed toward determining whether 'G' was 'schizophrenic' or not. It was not possible for 'G' to be a quarter schizophrenic or nearly schizophrenic or partly schizophrenic – he was either schizophrenic or he was something else (including 'normal', not ill, or whatever). In my example it is clear that the question is settled by referring to 'G's' medication – quite a common way of settling everyday puzzles and ambiguities. Determining a diagnosis for someone was, of course, a far more complex business than is suggested here and was a process carried out by means of a wide array of organisational activities. What I would like to emphasise here, however, is that nurses and psychiatrists basically regarded illnesses as real categories. Patients were either 'suffering from' schizophrenia or from manic depression or from some other psychotic or neurotic disorder (and perhaps even from a mixture of such disorders), and the task of the professionals was seen in terms of bringing the patient through the illness into health and well-being.

In this respect, the decision as to what is and what is not a case of illness in a hospital is determined in an entirely different ideological frame from that which operates in research settings. For example, when we read Brown and Harris's (1978) study of the social origins of depression in women we can see that for inclusion in the main sample of 114 psychiatric cases, treatment and identification by psychiatrists was a *sine qua non* of selection. In the community sample, however, caseness was bestowed on subjects solely by using responses to a validated instrument – namely the PSE. In much the same way, the Meltzer *et al.* (1995) study used the CIS-R as the appropriate instrument – an instrument deliberately adapted so that lay interviewers could make judgements about psychiatric disorder.

Now when we examine the logic that lies behind the use of these instruments we can determine that they rest on a markedly different theory of illness to that which I have referred to above. In fact, the PSE involves an interview schedule and scored responses so that the interviewer ends up with a numerical score rather than a diagnosis. From the Midtown Manhattan Study (Srole *et al.* 1962) onward, most studies of psychiatric morbidity in the community have used similar instruments wherein the resultant scores can be statistically manipulated to develop varying and emergent patterns of disorder. More significantly, this emphasis on scores can be said to reflect a very different concept of disease or illness from that which persists in the hospital. Indeed, it is a very different concept from that which dominated psychiatric work during the first half of the twentieth century in general. For during that period it was firmly argued that diseases – as discrete entities – truly existed and that a given individual either showed evidence of a diseased mind or not. For various reasons, however, (Armstrong 1983, Prior 1993) this ontological vision of disease had collapsed by the century's mid-point and in its place arose a vision of disease as a quantitative variation on the normal. In other words medicine began to embrace an image of disease and health as idealised states sited at the opposite ends of a finely graded continuum. In the routine course of everyday life, individuals were rarely to be considered diseased or healthy but as tending toward one or other of the two states; and the extent to which an individual tended towards disorder or 'normality' could be measured by the use of any one of a number of suitably constructed scales. As such we might say that the use of scaling techniques reflects a distinctly modern – 'quantitative' – vision of disease. It was this quantitative understanding of disease – inspired by the work of Adolf Meyer – that underpinned the nosology contained in the first and second editions of the *Diagnostic and Statistical Manual* of the American Psychiatric Association. Furthermore, it was this under-standing that ousted the older Kraepelian notions of distinct and iden-tifiable psychiatric diseases off the psychiatric map.

Given the quantitative theory of disease, then, it is clear that the identification of cases of psychiatric disorder in community surveys is ultimately dependent on the recognition of a score – a cut-off point or threshold – and not simply upon any quality buried deep within the human subject. So in that sense we can have as many or as few cases as we wish in any given study. Indeed, as Wing *et al.* (1981: 5) argued, 'It is clear that no single definition of a "case" can be given which is applic-able to all community samples'. For what is and what is not to be con-sidered a case depends very much on the aims and purposes of a study.

It is, of course, on grounds such as these that psychiatric epidemi-ologists are able to give emphasis to the socially constructed nature of cases. Indeed, Copeland moves so far as to argue that, 'The concept of case is a chimera existing only in the mind of the investigator' (1981: 11). However, in this chapter it is argued that the concept of case exists only in and through the mutual social relations and resultant social practices of researchers, psychiatrists, social workers, psychiatric nurses and the like. For it is truly through the maelstrom of social action that cases are manufactured. There has been a broad tendency in psychiatric epidemiology to argue that the identification of cases is to be regarded, in the main, as a technical operation. That is, an operation dependent solely upon the use of instruments and specialised psychiatric expertise. Though followed through to a logical conclusion such a position further suggests the possibility of regarding rates of psychiatric disorder as the product of the very instruments which measure that rate. Let us look at a few examples of this process.

Brown (1981), in a discussion of his study, provides a table in which case prevalence is defined according to three different sets of criteria. The percentage of 'cases' in the Camberwell study ranges from 11% to 21%, depending on the cut-off points which are used in the scoring system. And as Brown himself points out, the division between cases and borderline cases is crucial because the etiologic significance of social factors depends precisely on which cases are to be included and which are to be excluded. In other words, the decision as to where to place the cut-off point is dependent on organisational concerns, (in this instance, the concerns of a research organisation), rather than on any naturally occurring data in the community.

The same problems arise in the OPCS study mentioned above where the overall threshold score for 'significant psychiatric morbidity' was set as a score of 12 on the CIS-R. This particular score could, of course, be composed of responses drawn from all sections of the general instrument and in that sense does not result in a diagnosis *per se*. To obtain a diagnosis an algorithm is used so as to combine and recombine scores from the CIS-R, and such practices are, of course, entirely legitimate. What is important to note, however, is that subjects can often form the basis for any one of a number of diagnoses – psychiatric cases do not come ready wrapped for researchers. Consequently in any survey of the kind being discussed, rules of hierarchy and precedence have to be established so as to place the subject into one (and only one) appropriate box. In the case of the OPCS study, for example, subjects showing signs of the functional psychoses and other and milder neurotic disorders would have been given the diagnosis relating to psychosis. Subjects showing evidence for a diagnosis of generalised anxiety disorder (GAD) and a depressive disorder would have classified according to the depressive episode. Though GAD, in turn, would have taken precedence over a panic disorder and so on. In short, then, cases of both mild and severe mental illness (SMI) have ultimately to be defined in terms of research criteria.

Finally, one has to recognise the impact of the time variable on all of these deliberations. For, whatever instrument or scales we use, we must be aware that in the context of a morbidity survey, any given individual only constitutes a case in the relatively short time-frame of the research. A person is a case now, but may not have been 12 months ago or may not be a case 3 months into the future. In that sense the case is always current and fleeting. Only in the context of practical psychiatric work are psychiatric disorders likely to be associated with lifelong personal identities.

So far, I have talked about the construction of cases by researchers but researchers deconstruct cases as often as they construct them. We have to recognise that in much of social scientific research the case is not simply constructed and assembled according to research needs and research interests, but also disassembled and dissolved into a flux of variables. This is plainly so in what we might call survey research, where what researchers are interested in is not so much the personal bio-graphical detail of the case as a human subject, but the human subject as a bearer of key variables such as class, gender, ethnicity or whatever. Thus the 'case' (qua person) may come to be viewed as nothing more nor less than the embodiment or interstices of a set of social variables or as carriers of life 'events' and so on. Indeed, as Abbott (1992: 62) has argued, in a big survey research we often witness 'a narrative of acting variables' rather than a narrative of acting individuals. So that, 'Cases are characterless; they have no qualities other than those hypothesized to determine the dependent variable, and even those qualities act in iso-lation from one another.' (1992: 62). Thus in Brown and Harris' 1978 study, while their report provides a great deal of discussion concerning, say, personal life events, ultimately it is variables that are being exam-ined rather than people. In fact, the subject is of interest only in so far as she exemplifies the operation of the variables, and what any given individual is a case of alters and changes throughout the research. Here the subject is a case of depression, there a case of working class womanhood.

Cases and subjects, then, are inextricably interwoven, but researchers only take out of subjects what concerns them as cases. In that sense cases are always created or constructed – albeit constructed according to the demands of a research programme. Equally, however, cases are frequently deconstructed or disassembled such that research operations and research reports provide us with a narrative of variables rather than a narrative of acting subjects. In this respect, the subject is more often than not dissolved into the collective for the purpose of research operations and only later reconstructed for the purposes of a report. This is especially obvious when one considers the use of probability assess-ments or odds-ratios (e.g. Meltzer *et al.* 1995). For probabilities, by their nature, can only be derived from the study of collectives yet in research reports inevitably they are pinned on to individuals so as to create an impression that we can talk about the probabilities of *this* woman or *this* man experiencing a psychiatric episode, or whatever (Prior 1995). Underlying all of these processes is the tendency to argue that the recognition of cases is primarily a technical procedure that can be executed with the use of validated research instruments. That is to say, a belief that given the correct instrument we can recognise a case when we see it, for caseness is a property of persons rather than of organi-sations and with an accurate focus, a case can always be identified.

Cases as products of everyday professional practice

To Foucault the entire concept of a case belongs to, and emerges out of, a specific historical juncture (1977: 184). Foucault consistently argued that the 'case' could only be considered in terms of the professional practices which surrounded it and the institutional base of its production (1995: 792). This was so whether we were to consider cases in medicine, psychiatry, penology or pedagogy. Consequently he regarded it as erroneous to consider caseness a property of individuals. On the contrary, cases were necessarily products of wider and collective discursive practices.

In this section I consider caseness specifically in the context of organisational needs and organisational practices. To that end I begin with an observation offered by Strauss *et al.* (1963), to the effect that when people work together they commonly 'negotiate an order'. For the most part, that order serves to define lines of responsibility, authority and professional liability. It will also define, in various ways, who is to be regarded as competent to pronounce on this or that issue of practice. It will provide a 'bank' or store of rules and precedents in terms of which everyday organisational decisions may be made, in addition to rules and decisions about resource allocation and so on. Understandably, it is normally in terms of such rules and associated world views that decisions affecting caseness will be made. Yet, no matter how systematic any rule system might be made, there will always be a multiplicity of interpretations available as to how the regulations and standards specified in the system should apply to *this* person or to this particular case.

The presence of an 'order' does not, of course, preclude the possibility of conflict. For there are always periods in organisational life when the stability and legitimacy of the work order are questioned and queried by the individuals engaged within it. So in recent years, for example, there have been contests and clashes in the world of psychiatry about who can determine what is and what is not a suitable case of psychiatric disorder for professional intervention (Griffiths 1997). And in this respect psychiatrists have had to find ways of handling their monopoly on diagnosis in the broader framework of work in a psychiatric team composed of social workers and community psychiatric nurses as well as of medically trained psychiatrists.

For almost any psychiatric team there will exist, somewhere, an official and public statement about the objectives of the service being offered. In most cases those objectives will be stated in terms of such things as the 'needs' or requirements of subjects as clients of the organisation. There are also likely to be formally agreed procedures for screening and for assessing clients and their needs, as well as statements about how such needs might be met. Indeed, in the late twentieth century world of community care, 'needs-led assessment' procedures are common.

Discussions on needs-led assessments, of course, always imply that it is the qualities (or perhaps even the lack of certain qualities) in the subject which drives the assessment. In other words, it is implied that when clients are screened or assessed, the decision as to whether the client is entered on to the registers of the organisation depends solely on the properties, characteristics and circumstances of the clients themselves. Yet *all* such assessments are also made in the context of knowledge concerning organisational need. For example, in their discussion of needs-led assessments in social service settings, Lewis & Glennerster (1996) point out how some (untrained) social workers seemed to have difficulty thinking about need rather than services. In other words social workers would think about what services were available and then view the need of the individual in terms of available organisational resources – for residential care say. Indeed in one of their examples, they suggest that it was organisational need (of a hospital for a bed) which formed the occasion for what one care manager called 'a final flourish of assessment' (1996: 154) and which resulted in the discharge of the patient. Lewis and Glennerster discuss such instances in the light of bad practice, or in terms of aberrations and professional oversight. In what follows, however, I shall suggest that their examples of what might be called organisational primacy (as against client primacy) are far from constituting mere aberrations and deviant cases. Instead, they should be more properly seen as illustrative of (a) the routine ways in which organisations relate to subjects as cases, and (b) the ways in which organisations relate to people as subjects.

In my study of hospitalised psychiatric patients (Prior 1993) I noted how persons as clients were routinely disassembled for organisational purposes. As a sociologist, I found it intriguing that one and the same person could have any number of separate case notes and case histories associated with them, depending upon the kinds of professionals with whom they came in contact. Thus a psychiatrist might write up a 'chart' or medical notes and place such notes in one office. The nurses might write up the nursing care notes – covering all manner of things not dealt with in the aforementioned chart – and lodge them in the ward office. The social workers might inscribe a third set of notes on patients and lodge them in a third set of offices, and for some individuals there might also be legal and criminal records to consider. Even within the separate documents one could see a further fracturing at work wherein the subject was described under such headings as 'history', 'appearance', 'behaviour' and so on. The person as a subject was in that sense fragmented and fractured according to different organisational concerns and requirements – even though the subject as client was supposedly to be dealt with as a unity. In most instances, the various observations on the subject as a client were brought together at the team meeting, but this was not always so. For example, social workers in particular, were keen to preserve certain kinds of information as confidential and privileged and therefore reluctant to divulge all details of a case to nurses. In any event the 'team' served to manage the case rather to define it – definition was a process left to the various professions.

More importantly, it was evident to me that the way in which subjects were described and assessed by the professionals with whom they came in contact depended, not so much on some secret inner qualities which 'clients' may or may not have possessed (such as a disturbed personality or whatever), but rather on how the organisation could relate to them. For example, for some years and decades previous to my study the majority of patients had been considered as weak and vulnerable, as lacking insight into their disorders, as lacking in the social skills necessary for an independent life, as ill, and sometimes as unruly and disordered. During my period of study and for the majority of patients, the probability of each one of these kinds of assessments being over-turned improved markedly. However, it was not so much that patients had suddenly 'got better' or more skilled in daily living practices and social relations; nor had they become less disturbed, or gained greater insight into their psychiatric condition. In fact, as far as the majority of subjects were concerned, things were much the same. What did change were the number of organisational openings for 'independent' or community living. As more openings appeared, more and more assessments were made concerning the capacity for independence. This was so although detailed psychological assessments carried out some two years before my study had 'found' that only a tiny minority of the hospital population were capable of independent living.

Such reassessments and reinterpretation of subjects as cases are common enough in psychiatric organisations. In fact, my attention was first drawn to the myriad ways in which clients are defined and redefined according to organisational need from a reading of Byrd's (1981) study of an outpatient clinic. However, to illustrate in some detail how organisations both fragment and define clients as subjects in accordance with organisational rather than personal concerns I shall refer to two particular cases, both constructed in retrospect. The process of their construction was detailed and meticulous, though that was so simply because they involve histories of deviant and violent acts. Their utility for us rests on the fact that they are published case histories. At the practical level these case histories serve us as data. At a more fundamental and human level they provide a set of warnings about what happens when the needs of specific individuals fail to mesh with available organisational openings.

On 17 December 1992, Christopher Clunis murdered Jonathan Zito in a London train station. This, and other events, formed the occasion for an inquiry (Ritchie *et al.* 1994). It was only in and through that inquiry that Clunis as a 'case' with a long and convoluted history was constructed. Indeed, in some ways one might say that a key finding of the inquiry was that the failure ever to consider Clunis as a single, identifiable subject led to the tragedy of December 1992.

From 1986 onward it seems that Clunis was variously diagnosed as having paranoid schizophrenia, schizophrenia with negative features, drug-induced psychosis, a transient psychotic state, schizoaffective illness and so on. He was also observed to be violent, and sexually familiar and disinhibited with strangers. Between June 1987 and March 1988 alone, he was admitted to hospital six times and during subsequent years the number of admissions multiplied. He also came in contact with the police for various misdemeanours such as stealing sweets, but invariably was diverted away from the criminal justice system and towards the psychiatric system. This failure by the police to treat him as a priority case for prosecution seemed to have persisted even when more serious offences involving violence occurred. In short, he was not considered a case for the police. Yet, nor was the psychiatric system ready to embrace him wholeheartedly. In fact, admissions to hospital were usually short-term and he was more often than not diverted toward hostels, and agencies for the homeless on the grounds that his violent and aggressive behaviour constituted a risk to patients and staff. The Report (Ritchie *et al.* 1994) variously comments how his discharge from hospital had often taken 'precedence over his health and well being' (p. 16) – that is, his needs – and how lack of resources encouraged hospitals not to admit him or encouraged them to be rid of him as soon as possible (p. 43). Consequently, he was often 'treated as a single, homeless, itinerant' (p. 8), rather than as someone in need of close medical supervision – except when he was 'sectioned' under the Mental Health Act. Furthermore, professionals from different groups failed to share information about Clunis, and sometimes hid information (about his violence). His contact with social workers was fleeting and transient. The geographical boundaries of London were, it appears, used to shift responsibility for Clunis from one borough to another; and at one crucial point in his career it was claimed that he was 'capable of self-care and should be able to cope with independent living' (p. 83). A written judgement that there was no 'need for social work intervention' (p. 83), further ensured an absence of contact between Clunis and the social services. Thus, it appears, he was not a case for social work intervention either. In addition, the Report makes reference to the fact that close to the time of the murder, his GP removed him from his list – so neither was he considered a suitable case for general practice.

Indeed, what the Report documents is that Clunis as a subject was fractured and subdivided in accordance with the needs and aims of separate organisational entities, rather than his own personal needs as a subject. Thus, each episode of care was treated in isolation from the others, and consequently he became one of many cases/clients in different organisations at different times. His aggression and violence ensured that medical and other agencies would attempt to redefine his needs so as to free him from a given sphere of operations. In the words of the Report, 'there was a tendency to postpone decisions or action when difficulty was encountered, or perhaps because the patient was threatening and intimidating, and possibly because he was big and black' (p. 107). Indeed, both geographical and organisational boundaries were used so as to redefine needs and problems. Moreover, it is clear that all the signs and symptoms displayed by Clunis between 1987 and 1992 did not add up to a professional case for care and treatment in the absence of an explicit organisational decision or recognition to embrace him as such.

Similar features appear in my second example which is no less tragic, and certainly far more sordid. It concerns a Shaun Anthony Armstrong who raped and murdered 4-year-old Rosie Palmer during the summer of 1994. Once again, Armstrong was only ever considered a single, undifferentiated and identifiable case in retrospect and once again it was the published Report (Freeman *et al.* 1996) that provided the imprimatur of caseness.

Among other things the Report of inquiry into Armstrong's behaviour illustrates how, during the 1980s and 1990s, he moved almost effortlessly between the criminal justice system and the world of psychiatric hospitals and wards. He was variously diagnosed and described as suffering from depression, of being dependent on drugs and alcohol and of having a personality disorder and a psychopathic personality. He was also fined and imprisoned for various offences and had been investigated in relation to sexual offences. Interestingly the Report only manages to disentangle the multiple points of contact between Armstrong and the psychiatric and criminal system by narrating his biography in terms of organisational sequences – so his biography was written in terms of organisational contexts.

Armstrong as a client and as a subject was formally described, accounted for and referred to in various registers – social services registers, probation registers, registers concerning child sexual abuse, police registers, in-patient and out-patient registers. Yet, the exchange of information on Armstrong as a single autonomous subject was limited to the extent that no agency ever 'looked at the totality of the case' (p. 88). Each criminal and medical episode in his life was therefore investigated and dealt with on an isolated basis (p. 88), and there was little communication of information between agencies. For the most part, Armstrong was seen as 'a housing problem' – a problem that had only tangential relevance for the psychiatric professionals. On at least one occasion, his relationship to psychiatric facilities was defined away on the basis that, 'there were no tablets which could be given to him to resolve his problems' (p. 57). In other words, because he had no treatable mental illness, the psychiatric unit as a medical organisation excluded him from consideration. In a similar way the social services agencies had excluded him from consideration because he apparently failed to meet the criteria set for the implementation of the Care Programme Approach. The latter was only implemented under certain conditions (such as the presence of three or more admissions to hospital within a twelve-month period). And it was here that he was viewed primarily as a housing problem (the housing department, however, accepted him as a suitable case for housing only on grounds of his 'vulnerability' as defined by a consultant psychiatrist).

In line with this fragmentation, Armstrong had numerous histories – written up by different people working in different agencies. The Report's authors in fact criticise the paucity of history taking in both nursing and social work and especially the manner in which hospital nurses had described Armstrong in terms of a specific model that had been designed for use in the hospital as a whole and which was unsuitable for use with psychiatric patients. Nevertheless, nurses had variously described Armstrong as '(p. 1) pleasant and sociable ... (p. 9) tall with glasses ... (p. 12) wearing Cuban heels ... (p. 13) slimy (p. 14) a story teller' (p. 74). Not being in receipt of psychotropic medication, however, Armstrong was not truly considered as a case of mental illness, (cf. my own example that opened section 'Cases as products of technical procedures').

In summary then, Armstrong was not in any sense considered a case for hospital treatment or for care management because he did not fit in with the mission statements and screening processes of the various organisations with which he came in contact. Each organisation had confronted him in terms of its specific and limited organisational procedures, and there had been a failure of agencies to share information on him as a person. To become a case for care or treatment he would, of course, have had to have been manufactured as a case – in much the same way as the Consultant Psychiatrist had manufactured him as a case of someone who was vulnerable and homeless. It was never likely that Armstrong's caseness would simply unfold as a feature of some inner, secret self. Whether his recognition as a case would have prevented the murder, however, can only ever be a matter for speculation.

The Reports on Clunis and Armstrong illustrate, then, a number of key findings about the practical nature of caseness. First, it is clear that no technical instrument alone could identify those individuals as cases – for caseness is never a matter of imminent technical discovery. So when attempts were made to use a screening instrument on Armstrong and even on Clunis, each individual was regarded as falling outside of the stated criteria – presumably because the screening instruments were devised so as to fit organisational needs rather than the needs of clients. (Not surprisingly, the aggressive, violent, and difficult-to-deal-with are very often screened out from organisational territory). Second, it is clear that neither Armstrong nor Clunis were regarded as 'naturally occurring' cases. On the contrary they did not present themselves as cases for detention, care management or even for housing, but had to be constituted as such through the manipulation of bureaucratic procedures. Clearly, the criteria for caseness were not to be found within them as isolated subjects. Third, the organisational arrangements actually fractured them as subjects and ignored them as persons. Each person was constituted as a case only in retrospect, and their status as subjects was constituted only through the social and organisational relations which impinged on their lives. In short, both their caseness and their qualities as subjects were derived through organisational procedures rather than from their personhood.

Conclusion: the social construction of cases

Social constructionist arguments in the realm of medical sociology and the sociology of science can often call forth strong criticism (Bury 1987, Weinberg 1996); and there can be little doubt that the challenge which constructionist arguments pose to belief in the steadfast facticity of world generates both ideological and epistemological problems. In this chapter, however, I hope that I have gone some way to illustrating how considerations concerning the ways in which 'cases' are socially constructed through social and organisational relationships can have useful and fundamental practical application. For, from a sociological standpoint, it is possible to argue that it was failure to recognise the manufactured nature of caseness that contributed to the tragedies discussed above.

Cases, like all phenomena, simply are not 'natural kinds', and subjects rarely present themselves to agencies as ready-wrapped and defined phenomena. Even in those circumstances when subjects do self-define, as with entry to Alcoholics Anonymous, their self-labelling has still to be verified through social processes. Nor does the inner and secret self of the subject unfold to reveal illness, risk or danger. Such qualities as these have to be imputed and they are routinely so imputed in accordance with many tried and tested routines and social procedures. To that extent, a social science predicated on studying the secret impressions enveloped in an individual subject is destined to error. Among the routines and procedures to be studied we must count consideration of organisational needs and resources. In particular we must be aware that subjects as clients are routinely categorised and defined in terms of organisational activities. Each organisation will define the subject in accordance with its charter and will relate to such a subject only in terms of its charter. Moreover, an organisation will only relate to a subject in so far as it believes that it can offer a suitable organisational opening for the subject as a client. Hence, the refusal of a welfare agency or of a psychiatric agency to embrace a given subject, or a refusal by an agency to incorporate the subject into its realm of activities does not necessarily mean that the subject has no psychiatric problems, it merely implies that the organisation has no ready means for responding to them.

References

Abbott, A. (1992) What do cases do? Some notes on activity in sociological analysis. In: *What is a Case? Exploring the Foundations of Social Inquiry* (eds C.C. Ragin & H.S. Becker), pp. 53–82. Cambridge University Press, Cambridge.

Armstrong, D. (1983) *The Political Anatomy of the Body*. Cambridge University Press, London.

Barrett, R. (1996) *The Psychiatric Team and the Social Definition of Schizophrenia. An Anthropological Study of Person and Illness*. Cambridge University Press, London.

Brown, G. (1981) Etiological studies and the definition of a case. In: *What is a Case? The Problem of Definition in Psychiatric Community Surveys* (eds J.K. Wing, P. Bebbington & L.N. Robins), pp. 62–9. Grant McIntyre, London.

Brown, G. & Harris, T. (1978) *Social Origins of Depression. A Study of Psychiatric Disorder in Women*. Tavistock, London.

Bury, M.R. (1987) Social constructionism and medical sociology: a rejoinder to Nicolson and McLaughlin. *Sociology of Health and Illness*, **9**, 439–41.

Byrd, D.E. (1981) *Organizational Constraints on Psychiatric Treatment: The Outpatient Clinic*. JAI Press, Greenwich.

Copeland, J. (1981) What is a 'case'? A case for what? In: *What is a Case? The*

Problem of Definition in Psychiatric Community Surveys (eds J.K. Wing, P. Bebbington & L.N. Robins), pp. 9–11. Grant McIntyre, London.

Foucault, M. (1977) *Discipline and Punish*. Penguin, Harmondsworth.

Foucault, M. (1995) *Dits et ecrits*, Vol. III. Gallimard, Paris.

Freeman, C.J., Brown, A., Dunleavy, D. & Graham, F. (1996) *The report of the inquiry into the care and treatment of Shaun Anthony Armstrong*, Tees District Health Authority, Middlesborough.

Griffiths, L. (1997) Accomplishing team: Teamwork and categorisation in two mental health teams. *Sociological Review*, **45**, 59–78.

Lewis, J. & Glennerster, H. (1996) *Implementing the New Community Care*. Open University Press, Buckingham.

Lewis, G. & Pelosi, A.J. (1990) *Manual of the Revised Clinical Interview Schedule*, (CIS-R). Institute of Psychiatry, London.

Meltzer, H., Gill, B., Petticrew, M. & Hinds, K. (1995) *The Prevalence of Psychiatric Morbidity among Adults living in Private Households*. OPCS Surveys of Psychiatric Morbidity in Great Britain, Report 1. HMSO, London.

Prior, L. (1993) *The Social Organization of Mental Illness*. Sage, London.

Prior, L. (1995) Chance and modernity. Accidents as a public health problem. In: *The Sociology of Health Promotion* (eds R. Bunton, S. Nettleton & R. Burrows), pp. 133–44. Routledge, London.

Ragin, C.C. (1992) 'Casing' and the process of social inquiry'. In: *What is a Case? Exploring the Foundations of Social Inquiry* (eds C.C. Ragin & H.S. Becker), pp. 217–26. Cambridge University Press, Cambridge.

Ritchie, J.H., Dick, D. & Lingham, R. (1994) *The report of the inquiry into the care and treatment of Christopher Clunis*. HMSO, London.

Srole, L., Langner, T.S., Michael, S.T., Kirkpatrick, P., Opler, M.K. & Rennie, T.A.C. (1962) *Mental Health in the Metropolis: The Midtown Manhattan Study*. McGraw-Hill, New York.

Strauss, A., Schatzman, L., Ehrlich, D., Bucher, R. & Sabshin, M. (1963) The hospital as a negotiated order. In: *The Hospital in Modern Society* (ed. E. Freidson). Free Press, New York.

Walton, J. (1992) Making the theoretical case. In: *What is a Case? Exploring the Foundations of Social Inquiry* (eds C.C. Ragin & H.S. Becker), pp. 121–37. Cambridge University Press, Cambridge.

Weinberg, S. (1996) Sokal's hoax. *New York Review of Books*, **43**:13:11–15, and **43**:15:54–5.

White, C.H. (1992) Cases for identity, for explanation or for control. In: *What is a Case? Exploring the Foundations of Social Inquiry* (eds C.C. Ragin & H.S. Becker), pp. 83–104. Cambridge University Press, Cambridge.

Wing, J.K., Bebbington, P. & Robins, L.N. (eds) (1981) *What is a Case? The Problem of Definition in Psychiatric Community Surveys*. Grant McIntyre, London.

Chapter 3
Asking Questions in Social Research: Theory and Method

Steve Taylor and Nick Tilley

Introduction

Theory and method are inextricably intertwined in social research. Whether theory is acknowledged or not, 'pure' research is impossible. The very act of doing research will involve making certain contested assumptions about the nature of social reality and the way it is to be understood. This chapter examines the relation between theory and method in the sociological interview. We begin by outlining the theoretical traditions of positivism, interpretivism and realism. Next, we consider some of their implications for undertaking sociological research generally and asking questions in particular. We then illustrate some of the possibilities of the 'realist interview' by using the example of asking questions about eating disorders.

Positivism

Positivism is open to a wide variety of definitions (Halfpenny 1982). However, it is generally seen as a philosophy of knowledge stemming from the writings of Hume and developed in social science by Comte and Mill. Positivism embodies an ontology of nominalism and phenomenalism, an epistemology arguing that the only certain knowledge comes from observation and experience and a belief in the unity of scientific method. Those using a positivist approach argue, or more often merely assume, that explanation can be built up inductively from the accumulation of statistical findings and well corroborated observations from which empirically testable hypotheses can be deduced. Positivism makes a clear distinction between 'theoretical' and 'observational' language. Hypotheses can only be tested by reference to observational categories which are (apparently) independent of the data. For example, a well-known positivist critique of Durkheim's famous study of suicide (1952) is that the theory was not really testable as Durkheim provided no clear 'operational' definition of the key concepts of egoism and anomie. Thus in their positivist adaptation of Durkheim, Gibbs and Martin (1964) operationalised the key concept of social integration in terms of the observable indicator of status integration. Individuals typically occupy a number of statuses and Gibbs and Martin hypothesised that the less these statuses overlapped in a population the higher will be its suicide rate. They argued that the status integration hypothesis could then be confirmed or falsified in a manner which was impossible in Durkheim's formulation.

Positivism leads a curious double life in sociology. In general text-books and specialist works on theory the central ideas of positivism, especially the notion that the empirical world can be directly observed, have been subjected to such a battery of criticism that the word has become used as an indictment. Indeed, it must sometimes seem to sociology students that positivism is little more than a dead horse periodically trundled out for up and coming theorists to find new ways of flogging. However, turning to journals devoted to empirical research in specialist areas of the social sciences we find the assumptions of positivism not only still alive, but flourishing more or less unquestioned beneath an array of brute facts, samples, indicators and statistical correlations. Certainly in the sociology of health and illness, positivist ideas underpin most of the work in many key areas, such as measurement of health and illness and attempts to operationalise the effects of class, deprivation and social support on health.

This paradox is partly a consequence of the unfortunate separation of 'theory' and 'research' in contemporary sociology. However, it is also due to the fact that much of the theoretical criticism of positivism in sociology not only had little to offer researchers in practical terms but often appeared to be ruling out the possibility of an empirically based sociology. For example, the ethnomethodological critique of 'conventional' sociology, which was popular in the 1970s, when taken to its logical – or rather illogical – conclusions, became a denial of the possibility of any rational knowledge of the social world, including that provided by ethnomethodology! (Pawson 1989, Layder 1994). Pawson (1989:17) has argued that the failure of critics of positivism to generate alternative empirical research strategies meant that: 'positivism having lost every single epistemological battle over the years seems to have won the war, certainly in terms of research effort and funding'.

Indeed, one fairly common response to familiar critical arguments about the viability of empirical, and particularly statistical, social research has been to suggest that more rather than less positivism is needed. For example, writing about researching health care, Najman *et al.* (1992: 42) argued that

'If errors of observation and measurement are a problem in social research, which they undoubtedly are, then methods which more tightly control the process of data collection appear a better response than methods which allow such a process to continue. On this point positivists appear to have the argument in their favour since they rely on replication and repeated hypothesis testing thus providing opportunities for the individual bias of researchers to be factored out.'

Interpretivism

The interpretive, phenomenological or hermeneutical tradition in social theory, which has its roots in the German idealism of Rickert, Dilthey and Weber, stresses the ontological and logical distinction between the natural and the human sciences. The fact that people engage in conscious, intentional activities and attach meanings to their actions means that human societies are essentially subjective realities. Human institutions cannot be divorced from the varied understanding that people – including sociologists – have of them. For interpretivists, this effectively rules out the possibility of an objective understanding of societies and the social sciences cannot be expected to discover invariant laws of human behaviour. Rather, their aim should be to try to make human experiences more intelligible by interpreting them in terms of the subjective intentions of actors. Thus the interpretivist critique of Durkheim's *Suicide* advanced by writers such as Douglas and Baechler does not concern itself with the difficulties of operationalising key concepts, but rather with the very idea of trying to explain suicide in terms of abstract social causes (Taylor 1990). Interpretivists argue that rather than examining the distribution of suicide and the various factors associated with it, the aim of sociology should be to examine what different cultures and subcultures mean by suicide, and how suicidal meanings are constructed in given situations.

Interpretive sociology favours ethnographic, qualitative methods which bring researchers as close as possible to the subjects of their studies. In the sociology of health and illness the division made by Dilthey between science's concern with matter and social science's concern with mind is reflected to some extent in the division made by some medical sociologists between disease and illness. While disease is the province of the objective sciences, social definitions and subjective experiences of illness are the legitimate concerns of sociology. In this context a great deal of interpretive sociological work has focused on what Gerhardt (1985) has called the 'stigma paradigm'; for example, studies of the application of illness labels, patient careers and the construction of illness identities.

The idealist, phenomenological elements of interpretive theory as applied to health and illness have been pushed much further in an alternative approach which has been rather loosely labelled as 'social constructionism'. This approach is less concerned with the alleged distinction between 'objective' science and 'subjective' social science because it holds that all knowledge is socially constructed. The theoretical assumptions behind this approach are almost an inversion of those of positivism. In positivism a real world of observational things is described by 'fictional' concepts. In social constructionism we can only know the world through the relativistic ideas we have about it. Thus the focus of inquiry, usually through documentary data, is the ideas – including 'expert' ideas – that different groups hold about health, illness or the body (Armstrong 1983).

Realism

Realism, like positivism and interpretivism, has been construed in a variety of different ways. Our concern here is with scientific realism (Pawson & Tilley 1997). This shares with positivism a concern with an objective, scientific understanding of society, but rejects the positivist view that scientific theories are derived from observation. Like social constructionists it rules out any idea of theory-free knowledge. However, this only rules out a scientific understanding of society if one accepts a positivist view of science. For the realist, scientific concepts are not derived from observation, but in terms of their relation to each other. The aim of scientific work is to uncover the underlying mechanisms that bring about observable regularities. The mechanisms that trigger events are seen to be real, though often unobservable, and will only be activated if the context provides for their operation. Thus, according to realists, science aims to explain observed regularities in terms of underlying mechanisms which are triggered in specific contexts. From this perspective the scientific experiment, for example, is not the passive observation of natural events, but the active construction of controlled contexts in which conjectured mechanisms will be activated to produce observable regularities.

Like positivism and interpretivism, the basic ideas of realism have a long legacy in sociology and some elements of realist theory can be found in the works of Marx and Durkheim. Although sociological orthodoxy locates Durkheim's *Suicide* in the positivist tradition, it has far more in common with realism, as Durkheim attempted to explain the observed relationship between suicide and various rates of external association in terms of the generating mechanism of real but invisible 'suicidogenic currents'. For Durkheim (1952: 311) these causal forces

'far from being directly cognisable, have on the contrary profound depths inaccessible to ordinary perception, to which we attain only gradually by devious and complicated paths like those employed by the sciences of the external world.'

The realist view of science developed from the criticism of logical positivism of the 1920s and 1930s which formed the basis for the empiricist view of science. Its significance for social science has been examined in the writings of the 'new realism', most notably in the work of Harre (1986), Bhaskar (1986), Layder (1990) and Archer (1995). Though realism sees the structure and logic of scientific explanation to be similar in all areas of inquiry, like interpretivism it acknowledges important differences between social and natural scientific research. First, the social world is an open system and the social contexts enabling or inhibiting the operation of causal mechanisms are subject to chronic and rapid social change. This severely limits the scope for prediction and generalisation in social science compared to natural science, which can operate under closed, experimental conditions. Second, the causal mechanisms in social life operate through the agency of situated subjects rather than mechanically through the working of objects and thus, in contrast to structuralism for example, this necessarily involves the attempt to understand subjects' definitions of their situations.

Realism, like positivism, also leads something of a double life in sociology. In the theoretical literature while positivism is a term of indictment, realism – with its promise of an non-empiricist science of society – has become something of a term of commendation. Just as there are few self-confessed positivists, there are few anti-realists. However, in contrast to positivism, there is very little evidence of realist ideas underpinning bodies of empirical research, and even discussion of the possibilities of realist theory for applied research are comparatively rare and comparatively recent (Layder 1993, Pawson 1989, Pawson & Tilley 1997, Sayer 1992). In short, while many people seem to approve of realist theory, no-one seems sure what to do with it. It is hardly surprising, therefore, that the few references to realism in the sociology of health and illness have been essentially speculative rather than empirically based (Taylor & Ashworth 1987, Porter & Ryan 1996). In the following section we look at some of the implications of the theoretical traditions outlined above for methods of interviewing in social research.

The interview: theory, purpose and method

Talking to people is one of the main ways in which sociologists try to find out about the social world and the theoretical traditions outlined above influence both the methods and the expressed purpose of the interview. There is a clear affinity between the positivist idea of an objective, empiricist science of society and the structured interview, which enables a large number of responses to be collected in a standardised form which can be quantified and, as in the natural sciences, the data are easily accessible to other researchers. As Hakim (1987: 48) observed, one of the main attractions of the survey, or questionnaire, is that, 'the methods and procedures used can be made visible and accessible to other parties ... so that the implementation as well as the overall research design can be assessed'.

Interpretivist sociologists have advanced a series of fairly well documented objections to the structured interview stemming from their theoretical position that the aim of sociology is to try to comprehend the meanings that people give to their actions. First, they argue that the structured questionnaire, with its standardised questions and pre-coded limited range of responses, cannot provide any authentic information about the way people 'really' think, feel and act. Second, they argue that even within its own limited terms of reference, the statistical data obtained in the survey are of little real value as there is no necessary correspondence between the researcher's question and its interpretation by respondents. For example, respondents can mean many different things when they tick that they 'strongly agree' with a statement. Thus in talking to people interpretivists favour informal, unstructured interviews which allow people to express themselves in their own words and are capable of accounting for a range of meanings.

There are, of course, many sociologists – particularly among those engaged in more or less full-time research – who have little time for such theoretical and methodological purity. Instead, they advocate a pluralist, horses for courses approach. De Vaus (1991: 335), for example, evaluating the role of the survey in social research, argues that:

'In the end, methodological pluralism is the desirable position. Surveys should only be used when they are the most appropriate method in a given context. A variety of data collection techniques ought to be employed and different units of analysis used. The method should suit the research problem rather than the problem being fitted to a set method.'

However, despite their differences, positivist, interpretivist and pluralist approaches to the interview have in common the view that it is the respondent and the respondent's views that are the subject matter of the interview. It is this taken for granted assumption about the subject of the interview that scientific realism questions. For the realist, as we have observed, all data are necessarily the product of the theoretical categories in terms of which they are collected and interpreted. The interview is no exception. There are no 'uncontaminated' subjects' views, they only come to us via the views of the researcher. Pawson (1989, 1996) calls this the imposition problem.

In the structured interview, the researcher's framework of concepts and ideas is imposed on the subject from the start. The researcher designs the questions and the range of answers, and typically the respondent is kept in the dark about the purpose of the questions. Respondents are typically asked to position themselves – usually unconditionally – in relation to the various alternatives furnished by the researcher by 'agreeing', 'disagreeing' and so on. The end result is that the data are structured solely in terms of the concepts and variables chosen by the researcher and only a fragment of the subjects' ideas are conveyed. For example, in their research on class and mobility, Marshall *et al.* (1988) use a questionnaire dominated by questions on class and thus impose on their respondents the contested idea that people's experiences are shaped by their class position.

In this context, interpretive researchers have compared the structured interview unfavourably with the unstructured conversational interview. It is argued that the latter, by allowing subjects to express themselves in their own words, presents a more authentic picture of the way things really are for them. For example, in their book on research methods for nurses, Sapsford & Abbot (1992: 32) appear to be in no doubt that: 'a definite strength of "open" approaches to research – just talking to people without imposing much structure on what is being collected – is the immediacy, the vivacity, the feeling of actually "being there".'

However, the idea of 'actually being there' is in some ways misleading in the sense that it implies that the researcher is merely a passive observer, simply reporting some unvarnished truth about how subjects really see something. In the unstructured interview an unseen imposition takes place after the event. From the mass of data created during unstructured interviews, the researcher inevitably makes a selection. In the final analysis it is the researcher who decides what matters and how

the items fit together. In the end it is the researcher making an interpretation, telling a story. What is reported in the book, or the academic
journal is not, and can never simply be what actually happened. Thus, for
example, as Pawson (1998) wryly observes, it is perhaps not surprising
that in her research on becoming a mother Oakley always seemed to find
'those epidural fearing, consultant wary, control seeking views which
resemble her own'.

These observations are not intended to imply anything like the blanket
criticism of structured and unstructured interview methods that fly back
and forth between advocates of positivist and interpretivist theories. Nor
are they to suggest the kind of midway, horses for courses compromise
put forward by pluralists. Rather, they merely suggest that the kind of
access to the real world assumed, or implied, by many researchers is an
impossibility as there will inevitably be an imposition of the researcher's
views on the data. One response to this is to suggest that the researcher's
theories should be 'up front' and out in the open rather than being, as it
were, smuggled into the research findings.

Given the central place that theory occupies in the realist view of
social science, a realist approach to the interview begins by recognising
that the interview is inevitably 'theory driven'. From this position
Pawson (1996) suggests we re-think the purpose of the interview. He
argues 'theorizing the interview' involves in the first instance a
recognition that it is not the respondent, but the researcher's theory that
is the subject matter of the interview, and 'the subject is there to confirm,
or falsify and, above all, to refine the theory'.

The realist has no specific commitment to any particular interview
technique. The point is that the researcher takes advantage of respondents' typical willingness to try to provide responses that are orientated
to the researcher's interests. A learning process can take place where the
respondent can learn what the researcher is interested in and shape their
replies accordingly. Thus, in the realist interview, the researcher has to
make the purpose of the question sufficiently clear for the respondent to
furnish a response that is orientated towards the needs of the researcher.
While respondents will clearly not know everything there is to know
about their own behaviour, what they are experts in – and what interviewers have always traded on – is their expertise on their own actions,
their views about the options available to them and their own way of
choosing between them. The interviewer needs to focus on what the
respondent is expert at and design the interview to tap that expertise.
The researcher uses that expertise in relation to those parts of the theory
to which it is relevant and the interview is thus openly driven by the
theory. The respondent needs to know enough of the researcher's concerns (defined by theory) to orientate the provision of responses

accordingly, in effect to teach the interviewer what is of relevance that they can know; that is, how they fit with the expectations of the theory about how they act, think and make choices in particular situations. The researcher can use the data as a basis for refining, refuting, corroborating, evaluating and arbitrating between theories. In the following section we look at an example of the realist interview taken from some of our current research.

The realist interview: an illustration

We used the realist interview in the course of on-going research into the 'illness careers' of a sample of young people with anorexia. Our intention is to examine explanations for the initial decision to change eating patterns, to continue restricting food intake to the point of self-starvation and, ultimately, to increase the amount eaten. We piloted realist interviews designed to arbitrate between and possibly refine some of the major theories of anorexia. Questions were devised which aimed at presenting the theories, so far as they relate to choice making, to the respondents, who were then asked to position themselves in relation to the theories' conjectures about their decision making. Of course, theories will normally refer to 'unacknowledged conditions' about which subjects will be unable to comment. The questions about decision making presented here relate to those aspects in the theories about which the respondent could be expected to have some expertise: their grounds for their food intake decisions. As Pawson (1998) suggests:

'(the realist interview) is not "hygienic research", nor a "transition to friendship", but a research relationship which allows respondents to think, "well, that's your theory but in my experience it happens like this".'

The pilot study referred to here consisted of extended interviews with 12 children, aged 11–16, who were living in a residential institution to which they had been brought because their apparently persistent and extreme determination not to eat had put their lives in jeopardy. Because of their youth it was decided that the best way in which to present them with theories of decision making was through short vignettes. Subjects were then asked to say whether they were just like the person in the story, nothing like them, quite like them or just a bit like them. They were also asked to elaborate on their replies. Respondents were given the full set of vignettes at the start of the interview to try to indicate that there was a range of possibilities. The research instrument is shown in the appendix to this chapter. Readers familiar with literature on anorexia will recognise the efforts to present some of the theories concerning decision making in a simplified and accessible form. For the purpose of illustration here we concentrate on the decision to reduce food intake and look at self-assessment in regard to decision making in terms of the (broadly sociological) theory of the 'social pressures' to be thin and the (broadly psychological) theory of the desire to exert control over one's life. However, our concern here is not with anorexia as such, or the variety of theories seeking to illuminate its origins, but with the interview. Also, with such a small sample and the research in its comparatively early stages, we are not seeking to advance anything that may be construed as a conclusion or even a finding, we are merely concerned here to illustrate a particular method of interviewing.

Social pressures

It is almost an orthodoxy in the sociological literature that anorexia is a pathological consequence of social pressures to be thin. Young women are particularly at risk because most of the pressure is placed on them and, indeed, it has been estimated that the ratio of females to males suffering from anorexia is between 15:1 and 20:1 (Button 1993). It has also been argued that females are especially vulnerable to social pressures because of the emphasis during female socialisation on 'passivity, compliance and selflessness'. Dissatisfaction with body shape is far higher among women than men and research has shown that dieting among young women is more prevalent than non-dieting (Polivy & Herman 1987). Thinness is associated with attractiveness. Content analysis of the media, for example of advertisements, beauty contests and so on has shown that the cultural ideal of slimness has increased in recent times. An obsession with diet can make young people, and girls and young women in particular, vulnerable to anorexia.

The opening vignette in relation to which our respondents were asked to position themselves and add comments was:

Q1. Julie started to lose weight because she felt she was the wrong shape to be attractive.

When respondents indicated that they were in some respect like Julie, they were presented with the following vignette:

Q1a. Julie has impression from friends, family, magazines and T.V. that to be liked or loved you have to be slim.

The social pressure theory, rather to our surprise, received only partial confirmation from our respondents. Three respondents confirmed that they were just like, or quite like Julie.

Subject A
Q1a Yes, I'm quite a lot like that. Yes, I can see that.
Q1b Yes, quite a lot like her. Everyone who was slim was popular and had a lot of friends.

Interestingly, our one male respondent, also corroborated the theory.

Subject B
Q1a Quite like him (John was substitute for Julie). I can relate to that. I wanted to be attractive to others. I never got on with girls that much. I'm quite small. I thought, 'If I can't change my height, I can change my weight'. It started off from there. I wanted attention from everyone. I was fed up with the same group of friends. I wanted to spread around. I did think I was fat, but not immensely fat.... I became ill because I wanted to be attractive.
Q1b Yes, quite like him then. But I'm not like that now. You come to realise people like you for what you are. It doesn't matter what size you are – five stone or thirty. At the time looks were everything. The thinner you are, the more friends you have. You lose a stone, you get another friend. I was bullied, called 'fatty' by my own friends. I thought that if I wasn't fat they'd like me again, so I wanted to lose a few more pounds.

Three respondents simply said that they were not like Julie at all, while the other six gave a more qualified corroboration. While they recognised the existence of the social pressures to be thin and thought it may influence others, they did not feel it was a major factor in their own decision. Some went on to offer alternative, or supplementary, explanations for their own decision.

Subject C
Q1a I suppose I was a bit like her, yes. At the start. But I think it was really a means of punishing myself because I couldn't accept myself for who I was, and I couldn't see myself for who I was. I couldn't see myself as other people saw me and I couldn't feel accepted.
Q1b Yes, in some ways. It's all appearance , isn't it? ... It must have an influence on people.... But I didn't think people wouldn't accept me. I think it was basically that I wasn't acceptable to myself.... By denying my body what it needed, I was inflicting punishment on myself.

Subject D
Q1a Not really. I just didn't like myself. Not just my shape. I didn't like me. I didn't think anyone would like me.
Q1b No, not really like her, because I always knew I was loved. But I thought if I lost weight it would make me happy, then I'd like myself more and I'd be able to get on with my life.

Control

An alternative, social psychological theory of anorexia, greatly influenced by the work of Bruch (1978) seems at first to contradict the social pressure theory. Instead of representing compliance to others' images and expectations of conformity to a socially established notion of the ideal body shape, anorexia is construed as an attempt by the sufferer to recover some control of their life in the face of all-pervasive demands by others. Again, females are more vulnerable in so far as it is believed that their behaviour is more likely to be monitored and controlled than boys. Therefore girls more typically need to find some area over which they can exert control. Anorexia becomes a private means of exerting that control: a form of closet deviance where the individual has some space for self expression.

The three vignettes through which control theory about their choices were put to respondents were as follows:

Q3. Julie started to lose weight because she felt that this was one area of her life where she could exert some control for herself. Everything else she did to please other people.

Supplementary questions were only put if there were some identification with the main statement.

Q3a. Julie felt she had little space for herself. At least she could control her body.
Q3b. Julie felt that members of her family were controlling her life.

With the exception of one respondent (who provided no support for any of the theories) all our respondents offered very clear and strong confirmation of the control thesis. While seven identified strongly with the idea that their families were controlling their lives at the time, in retrospect most of them went on to qualify that view.

Subject E
Q3 Yes, quite a lot like her. I did think I was doing things for everybody

else. Because they bossed me about a lot, I thought I wanted to do something for myself. So I was quite a lot like her. When I started to lose weight I felt I did have control because nobody could interfere or anything, because they didn't know, so it was something I could control.

Q3a A bit like her ... um ... I don't know.

Q3b Yes, a lot like her. My parents weren't really controlling, but at the time it felt like that. I felt I wasn't doing anything for myself.

Subject F

Q3 Yeah, mostly I did it for myself 'cause if I lost weight it would be me doing it and I would have control over it. Everything else was not controlled by me. I was doing it for my mum, my boyfriend, or like school work – I had to do it....

Q3a Yes.

Q3b My dad always tried to control my life. That used to aggravate. But he didn't really control, he tried to tell me what to do. But I'd never do it. That caused arguments. I didn't want him to have control.

Subject C

Q3 Yes. I can identify with that. I valued myself for my achievements.... When I went down with ME I wasn't able to achieve and it became very frustrating and I felt I'd lost what made me. Everything seemed to be going out of control.... I was seeing a psychiatrist.... Nothing seemed to be getting any better, so I felt I didn't have anything left. I had no control over what was happening, so it became a way of forming an identity or something. Being able to prove self worth to myself more than anything.... By having control.

Q3a I suppose so, yes. In the end for me it was also about self punishment. I got to enjoy hurting myself.

Q3b I don't know. I haven't really thought about that one a great deal ... but, perhaps, yes ...

Subject B

Q3 Yes. I'm like him (John) there. This is one thing you can control. I felt really low. Depressed. You can control what you eat. What you put in and what comes out and how much exercise you take.

Q3a I felt control slipping away from me.

Q3b Yes, I agree. My dad pushed me very hard and put me under a lot of pressure. I'm sixteen, I don't want to be stuck indoors. I wanted to be out enjoying myself.... They said, 'do whatever you like, but its your GCSEs'. It was a guilt thing.... 'You'll never do anything if you don't get GCSEs....' You feel better if you're controlling something and I could control my body. It's really good to take control.

It is not our intention, from such a small sample, to make any evaluation of competing theories. The questions and the extracts from
respondents' answers were employed merely to illustrate some of the
possibilities of a type of realist interview. Not only would evaluation of
and adjudication between competing theories require much more data, it
would also involve some consideration of the institutional contexts
which might influence the construction of such data. It is this issue we
consider in the final section.

The context of research and the construction of data

The children in our sample lived in a total institution. They enjoyed no
privacy; their behaviour was tightly regulated; their weight, food intake
and waste were very closely monitored. None of them had decided
willingly to resume eating. All were coerced. They faced a strict regime
and, without it, some would not have survived. Although some members
of staff were strongly disliked, the children recognised that they had
been placed in there for their own good.

One of the concerns of our research which, as we shall try to show, is
relevant to the interview data, is the examination of the impact of this
regime on the children's sense of identity and perception of their situation. In his classic study of total institutions, Goffman (1991) examined
the process by which inmates' sense of identity is broken down and
reconstructed within the confines of the institution. How, we wondered,
might this process manifest itself in our total institution?

The emaciated child inmates were, for the most part, curiously mature
in the way they talked. Some were heartbreaking to look at, with gaunt
faces and spindly legs. They seemed old beyond their years in the way
they spoke to us; in conversation most were fluent, confident and
socially accomplished. With eyes shut, instead of school-aged children,
you would imagine the speakers to be young, educated, introspective
adults, capable of standing back and commenting reflexively on their
selves. Although one or two had little to say for themselves, by and large
we were interacting with pathetic waifs who spoke like bright post-
graduates in the behavioural sciences.

It soon became clear to us that those who had been in the home for a
significant period of time – like Subject C who had been there for nearly
six months – had become very used to talking about themselves and
their condition. A lot of this had to do with their treatment programme. A
second part of the regime being followed by the children involved
regular therapy sessions. They would regularly talk through their condition and the circumstances leading up to it with the professional
workers who were there to help them. Unlike most of their age-peers

these children had been given the opportunity to talk regularly about themselves. They knew something odd had happened to them and that their therapists were helping them to make sense of it. Those who had been in the home for any length of time had the vocabulary for, and were in the habit of discussing their own selves. They were unselfconscious in talking about their self-consciousness.

In his acclaimed study of blindness Scott (1969) argued that blindness is a 'learned social role' and that various experts play a major part in helping to construct for their clients a blind identity. It seemed to us that something broadly similar may be happening to the anorectic children we observed and talked to. Therapy was providing the children not only with an explanation for their situation, but they were being socialised into their new identity. A number of comments made by the children either in answers to our interview questions or in general conversation with us were significant in this context.

'I didn't realise at the time, but I can see now that at the time you are trying to control.'
'I didn't know what was happening until I came here and the therapist sort of finalised it and everything.'
'At the time I didn't realise anything was wrong, until I got here and thought, 'Gosh, something must be wrong.'
(In answer to a question) 'Well, I'm not sure we haven't covered that in therapy yet.'

Because the children most able to elaborate on their answers had been in quite intense therapy for a long time, their interpretation of the conditions and circumstances leading up to it had been constructed in conversation with experts in anorexia. It seems our interviews were the end product of a process of circular reasoning where the ideas of the therapists were reproduced by subjects and then discovered in research (Figure 3.1).

In the case of our respondents, their life in a total institution, their intensive therapy and the fact that they have to do well to obtain privileges and eventual release seems to make them especially open to therapeutic suggestion. It could be this that explains the wide confirmation of the 'control theory' held by many psychologists. It is perhaps significant that one respondent who did not align herself with it – or any of the other theories – had only been in the institution for a few days. None of this is to say the control theory is 'wrong'. However, the findings from our pilot realist interviews may have reflected processes where the very theory being put to our respondents may have had a part to play in helping them give a retrospective meaning to their behaviour.

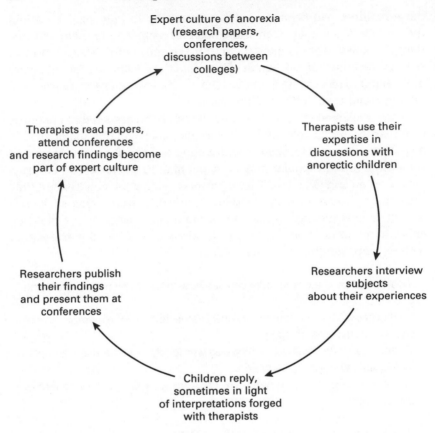

Fig. 3.1   The production of accounts of anorexia.

Conclusions

We have tried in this chapter to describe the ways in which different interview techniques are associated with differing theoretical traditions in sociology which are, in turn, derived from differing underlying philosophies of knowledge. We have focused on realism here because the powerful critique it makes of more familiar approaches of data collection in social research has been generally neglected in the sociology of health and illness. By presenting an example of some of the possibilities of realist interviewing drawn from research in progress, we have tried to highlight something of the distinctiveness of a realist approach. It has not been our intention to suggest that realism is somehow superior to other theoretical approaches. However, we have tried to show that it offers a distinctive way of defining and managing research problems, and we have suggested that sociological students of health could perhaps give scientific realism rather more consideration than they do at present. Finally, we have tried to show how in research on anorexia (and by implication other areas where people are subject to some form of expert therapy as a way of making sense of problems) researchers will face difficulties in constructing data which is not already influenced by the very theories that are being subjected to test and refinement.

References

Archer, M. (1995) *Realist Social Theory: The Morphogenic Approach*. Cambridge University Press, Cambridge.

Armstrong, D. (1983) *The Political Anatomy of the Body*. Cambridge University Press, Cambridge.

Bhaskar, R. (1986) *Scientific Realism and Human Emancipation*. Verso, London.

Bruch, H. (1978) *The Golden Cage: The Enigma of Anorexia Nervosa*. Routledge, London.

Button, E. (1993) *Eating Disorders: Personal Construct Therapy and Change*. Wiley, Chichester.

de Vaus, D. (1991) *Surveys in Social Research*, 3rd edn. Allen and Unwin, London.

Durkheim, E. (1952) *Suicide: A Study in Sociology*. Routledge, London.

Gerhardt, U. (1985) Stress and stigma explanations of illness. In: *Stress and Stigma: Explanation and Evidence in the Sociology of Crime and Illness* (eds U. Gerhardt & M. Wadsworth), pp. 161–204. Macmillan, Basingstoke.

Gibbs, J. & Martin, W. (1964) *Status Integration and Suicide*. University of Oregon Press, Eugene.

Goffman, E. (1991) *Asylums: Essays on the Social Situation of Mental Patients and other Inmates*. Penguin, London.

Hakim, C. (1987) *Research Design: Strategies and Choices in the Design of Social Research*. Allen and Unwin, London.

Halfpenny, P. (1982) *Positivism and Sociology: Explaining Social Life*. Allen and Unwin, London.

Harre, R. (1986) *Varieties of Realism*. Blackwell, Oxford.

Layder, D. (1990) *The Realist Image in Social Science*. Macmillan, London.

Layder, D. (1993) *New Strategies in Social Research*. Polity, Cambridge.

Layder, D. (1994) *Understanding Social Theory*. Sage, London.

Marshall, G., Newby, N., Rose, D. & Vogler, N. (1988) *Class in Modern Britain*. Hutchinson, London.

Najman, J., Morrison, J., Williams, G. & Andersen, J. (1992) Comparing alternative methodologies of social research: An overview. In: *Researching Health Care* (eds J. Daly, I. McDonald & E. Willis), pp. 138–57. Routledge, London.

Pawson, R. (1989) *A Measure for Measures: A Manifesto for Empirical Sociology*. Routledge, London.

Pawson, R. (1996) Theorizing the interview. *British Journal of Sociology*, **47**:2, 295–311.

Pawson, R. (forthcoming 1998) Research methods. In: *Contemporary Sociology* (ed. S. Taylor). Macmillan, Basingstoke.

Pawson, R. & Tilley, N. (1997) *Realistic Evaluation*. Sage, London.

Polivy, J. & Herman, C. (1987) Diagnosis and treatment of normal eating. *Journal of Consulting and Clinical Psychology*, **55**, 635–44.

Porter, S. & Ryan, S. (1996) Breaking the boundaries between nursing and sociology: A critical realist ethnography of the theory-practice gap. *Journal of Advanced Nursing*, **24**, 413–20.

Sapsford, R. & Abbott, P. (1992) *Research Methods for Nurses and the Caring Professions*. Open University Press, Buckingham.

Sayer, A. (1992) *Method in Social Science: A Realist Approach*, 2nd edn. Sage, London.

Scott, R. (1969) *The Making of Blind Men: A Study in Adult Socialization*. Russell Sage Foundation, New York.

Taylor, S. (1990) Suicide, Durkheim and sociology. In: *Current Concepts of Suicide* (ed. D. Lester), pp. 225–36. Charles Press, Philadelphia.

Taylor, S. & Ashworth, C. (1987) Durkheim and social realism: An approach to health and illness. In: *Sociological Theory and Medical Sociology* (ed. G. Scambler). Tavistock, London.

Appendix: Interview questions

I'm going to tell you some stories about a girl of your age. I want you to tell me in each case whether you are just like her, nothing like her, quite a lot like her or just a bit like her. Then I'd like you to tell me how you are like her or different from her. Let's call the girl Julie.

I'm going to start with a few stories about how Julie decided to try to lose weight.

1. Julie started to try and lose weight because she felt she was the wrong shape to be attractive.
1a. (If full or partial concurrence) Julie has the impression from friends, family and magazines that to be liked or loved you have to be slim.
2. Julie started to try and lose weight because she felt that it would be healthier to be slimmer.
2a. (If full or partial concurrence) Julie had picked up from health experts in magazines, friends and doctors that to be healthy you have to be slim.
3. Julie started to try to lose weight because she felt that this was one

area of her life where she could exert some control for herself. Everything else she did to please other people.

3a. Julie felt that she had little space for herself. At least she could control her body.

3b. Julie felt members of her family were controlling her life.

4. Julie started to lose weight because all boys and girls of her age like to be slim.

4b. (If full or partial concurrence) Julie's best friend was slimming and Julie wanted to be just like her.

Let me now turn to Julie's decision to carry on eating very little.

5. Julie still thinks she's thought fat and unattractive and therefore eats very little.

6. Julie continues to eat very little to stay healthy or to become healthier.

7. Julie continues to try to lose weight as a way of controlling her life.

8. Julie eats little just because she's not hungry any more.

9. Julie thinks she eats plenty of food for her own needs.

Finally, let me turn to Julie's decision to increase her food intake.

10. Julie has started to eat more because she thinks she's become unattractively thin.

11. Julie has started to eat more because she needs to do so to improve her health.

Chapter 4

Researching a Public Health Issue: Gay Men and AIDS

Mary Boulton, Ray Fitzpatrick and Graham Hart

Introduction

Sociological research, especially in areas such as health and illness, is increasingly carried out in response to problems defined by applied and policy driven concerns. Sociologists are expected to produce insights and explanations, less in order to satisfy the intellectual curiosity of the discipline and more to find solutions to problems. Yet once drawn into such applied work, the sociological challenges prove as fundamental and rewarding as any derived from classical sociological sources. There can be few more striking instances of this process than the research stimulated by the AIDS epidemic. Society was effectively ignorant of the social groups and social processes that, at an early stage, were implicated in the dynamics of the epidemic. Sociologists were called upon to use their expertise in investigating the social world in order to provide the insights essential to understanding and controlling the spread of the virus. In doing so, AIDS researchers have extended sociological knowledge and further developed theory and methods in the social sciences (Boulton 1993, 1994).

This chapter describes the methodological issues raised in a series of studies we conducted on the sexual behaviour of homosexual and bisexual men in relation to HIV and AIDS. From the beginning of the epidemic in the UK, unprotected sexual intercourse between men has constituted the most common route of HIV transmission and the sexual behaviour of homosexual and bisexual men has been of particular interest to those concerned with public health. Three linked studies are described here: two – the Gay Men's Health Studies – were large-scale quantitative studies; the third – Bisexual Men in Britain – was a small-scale qualitative study.

These two types of study illustrate different aspects of the contribution of sociology to public health generally and to the AIDS epidemic in particular. In the context of early anxiety about the spread of HIV and AIDS, accurate quantitative accounts of sexual behaviour were considered vital to enable health promotion services and the gay community to make informed decisions in their response to the epidemic. The Gay Men's Health Studies drew on the power of sociological survey methods for this purpose. At a later stage in the epidemic, a distinct moral panic arose regarding bisexual men as a threatening 'bridge' from gay men to the wider society. A qualitative study, Bisexual Men in Britain, examining the social reality of bisexuality was an equally important contribution of sociology, in this case to question a taken-for-granted epidemiological category and to challenge potentially damaging societal myths.

The gay men's health studies

In the context of the AIDS epidemic, a central concern of those involved in public health has been the development and evaluation of programmes to control and contain the spread of IIIV infection. Fundamental to this concern has been the need for accurate and up-to-date information about patterns of sexual behaviour in the population and for theories which can explain and predict the ways they are changing. Health promotion services, in particular, have required accurate accounts of sexual behaviour and an understanding of the factors that shape them, so that they can design effective interventions and target them appropriately.

Prior to the AIDS epidemic, however, little systematic research had been conducted on sexual behaviour in the UK and little attention had been paid to understanding the factors which influence it. This gave rise to an urgent need for research which could provide descriptions of sexual behaviour and explanations for variations in sexual behaviour, particularly among the population of homosexually active men where rates of HIV infection were highest. Our first two studies were undertaken to meet this need and were intended to provide the kind of information required for designing and evaluating health promotion interventions. The primary aims of the Gay Men's Health Studies were to describe the patterns of sexual behaviour amongst homosexual men – particularly the extent of unprotected anal intercourse which carries the highest risk of HIV transmission – and to identify the factors which promote or inhibit the adoption of safer sex practices – particularly the use of condoms in penetrative sex. In the first study, the Health Belief Model was used as the framework to identify processes which might explain variations in sexual behaviour in the context of the AIDS epidemic (Fitzpatrick *et al.* 1991). When this proved of limited value, a framework based on perceptions of partners and partner relationships was developed and tested in the second study (McLean *et al.* 1994).

Given the aims of the research, The Gay Men's Health Studies were conceived as large-scale, quantitative surveys. The reasons for this were quite straightforward. As a number of social scientists have argued, large-scale quantitative surveys allow researchers to test their theoretical propositions more rigorously and to generalise their findings more widely than would be possible with smaller, more interpretive studies (Marsh 1979, Bryman 1988). By 'measuring' key concepts in a large sample, we were able both to relate our descriptions of sexual behaviour to a wider population of homosexual men and to begin to tease out theories to explain why some men adopted safer sex practices and others did not.

The value of our research, however, turned on how well we managed to deal with two sets of methodological problems. The first concerns the representativeness of our samples; the second concerns the reliability and validity of the instruments we developed to measure our concepts. In the rest of this section, we will outline the particular challenges to sampling and measurement raised by research on sexual behaviour among homosexual men and the ways we tried to deal with them in our own work. By way of assessing how successful we were in dealing with them, we will also describe the characteristics of the sample we recruited and the extent of risky sexual behaviour they reported.

It is important to remember, however, that the study aimed not only to *describe* but also to *understand and explain* patterns of sexual behaviour. Although they will not be considered here, the development of instruments to measure the concepts central to our analytical frameworks – for example, perceived costs and benefits of adopting safer sex practices in the first study, and sexual attraction, trust and emotional commitment in the second – required as much care and attention as the development of instruments to measure sexual behaviour. By the same token, the efforts described in the following pages to establish the reliability and validity of our measures and the broad representativeness of our samples were important, not only to give confidence in the accuracy and relevance of our descriptions but also to give confidence in the rigour and precision with which we examined our theoretical propositions.

Research in a 'hidden' population: Recruiting a sample of men who have sex with men

Early in the AIDS epidemic, epidemiological research on the sexual behaviour of homosexual men had been conducted almost exclusively among men who attended genito-urinary medicine (GUM) clinics. These men were readily accessible to medical researchers and were well motivated to co-operate in research carried out in the clinics that provided their care. It became increasingly evident, however, that only a small proportion of homosexual men consulted GUM clinics and that those who did were unlikely to be typical of the population of men who have sex with men. Studies based on clinic samples were thus of limited value in estimating patterns of risky sexual behaviour in the wider population. Research needed to draw on more representative samples of homosexual men and it was clear that this would require recruiting men outside clinic settings, 'in the community'.

Recruiting men 'in the community', however, was much more problematic than recruiting men seeking treatment at a clinic. Despite the sexual revolution of the 1960s and burgeoning gay communities in many cities, homosexuality in the UK has remained a stigmatised and largely hidden activity (Weeks 1981). The emergence of the AIDS epidemic served only to increase attitudes of suspicion and hostility among large sections of the population, as the media created a moral panic out of what was presented as a 'gay plague'. Active discrimination against homosexuals increased and the gay community faced renewed threats from a wide range of sources. In these circumstances, it was generally expected that homosexual activity would be driven further underground: that men would be concerned to shield their homosexuality from public view and would be unwilling to take part in research which identified them in these terms.

Careful thought had to be given to the strategies we could use to identify and recruit men to our study. Of particular concern was recruiting a sample which would adequately represent the broad spectrum of men who had sex with men, rather than the more narrowly defined population of men who identified with the gay community. A statistically representative sample was never possible, as no reliable sampling frame of homosexual men existed from which a random sample could be drawn. Instead, the aim was to recruit as diverse a group of men as possible in order to try to include the full range of men who had sex with men. To maximise the diversity in our sample, we decided to conduct the study in several different geographical areas and to use several different strategies to locate and recruit men in each area.

In choosing the geographical areas to work in, we looked for places that were likely to offer different attractions to homosexual men. In the first study, we recruited men from four main areas: London and Manchester were chosen as national centres of the gay community in the north and south-east of England; Oxford and Northampton as smaller towns with more limited facilities for men who have sex with men. In the second study, we extended our efforts to include Bristol and Birmingham, as examples of cities in other regions of the country.

Because of the sensitivity of the research, in each of these areas considerable background work had to be done before any attempt could be made to recruit men for interview. It was particularly important to win the confidence of influential figures within the local gay community, whose support was important in gaining the trust of other men. The gay organisations in each area were contacted so that the aims and methods of the study could be explained. Members of the research team also explored the local 'gay scene' and represented the study to those active in this context. Finally, in each of the areas, the GUM clinics which were known to be used by gay men were approached and their co-operation and support obtained. By making the effort to work in partnership with the local community in this way, the research team was able to avoid the potential suspicion and resistance from homosexual men which would have made it impossible to carry out the study.

Efforts were also made to publicise the research so that potential respondents were familiar with the study before they were approached to take part in it. Members of the research team gave talks to community groups and political organisations about the research and, where it was requested, provided progress reports at subsequent meetings. Approaches were made to gay clubs and pubs for permission to put up posters and to allow distribution of leaflets within their premises. The study also attracted a certain amount of media attention. It was reported on favourably in the gay press nationally and, in some of the areas in which we worked, local radio stations ran interviews with members of the research team. Such 'positive talk' about the research helped to encourage men to volunteer for the study or to agree to take part in it when they were approached by a researcher.

Once the study was accepted in an area, a variety of strategies were used to recruit individual men for interview. Most important was what Lee (1993) calls 'outcropping' – finding sites where homosexual men congregated, and recruiting them from there. Since the emergence of the AIDS epidemic, researchers have shown considerable imagination and resourcefulness in identifying places where those involved in highly stigmatised or illegal activities gather (Boulton 1993). The sites we used included a large number of gay clubs, pubs and social centres. Individuals were approached in these sites and asked to take part in the study although those who agreed were generally interviewed at a later time and in a more appropriate place (e.g. their own home). The attraction of this strategy was the efficiency it afforded in quickly and easily recruiting large numbers of men who met the criteria for inclusion in the study. Its main drawback was in terms of the potential bias it introduced into the sample. Men attending particular pubs, clubs and organisations are unlikely to be representative of the wider population. Recruiting from a range of organisations helped overcome this bias to some extent, but men who did not use the facilities of the gay community were still missed out.

To extend recruitment outside the organised gay community and include those whose activities were more covert, we adopted a number of additional sampling strategies. GUM clinics provided recruitment sites which were not directly associated with the gay community and hence attracted a potentially different range of homosexually active men. Networking or 'snowball sampling' was also potentially useful although it proved less productive than expected. Because of the sensitive nature of the study, we did not approach the friends and associates of our participants directly but relied on them coming forward and contacting a member of the research team themselves. In the absence of external prompts, only a limited number of men did so.

Our final strategy was to place advertisements in the personal columns of several gay newspapers and in more widely read magazines such as *Time Out*. While the earlier media coverage had been intended to draw wide attention to the study and to present it in a positive light, these advertisements were intended to attract the attention of very specific categories of men, in particular those who were concerned to keep their homosexual activity hidden. While these men were less visible to the researchers, advertising could at least make the study more visible to them. However, while we felt we could reach the appropriate men through advertising, there was no guarantee that they would respond by getting in touch with a member of the research team. Advertising also ran the risk of attracting unwanted or inappropriate attention which could be difficult and distressing for the researchers to deal with.

Our criteria for inclusion in the study – that is, our operational definition of homosexual – was a man who had had sex with another man in the previous five years. This definition, based on behaviour and limited in time was essentially arbitrary and not inherently more 'accurate' than any other. It was, however, meaningful to the men with whom we were working and, in the context of our interest in HIV infection, it seemed most 'appropriate'.

Eventually, a total of 502 men were recruited to the first study and 677 to the second. In both studies, the samples were predominantly young (mean age 32 years, sd 10, range 16–71), white (over 90%) and middle class (first study 85%; second study 72%). The great majority (about 80%) also identified as 'gay'. Nevertheless, in both studies the samples represented a broad spectrum, including men of widely varying ages, education, occupations and income as well as men who did not identify as gay, men who were or had been married and men involved in a wide range of sexual activities (Fitzpatrick *et al.* 1990, Dawson *et al.* 1994).

In terms of their demographic characteristics, the samples in both studies resembled those recruited to other community studies carried out in Britain, North America and Australia (Connell *et al.* 1989, Joseph *et al.* 1987; SIGMA 1990). But while this might be considered encouraging evidence of successful sampling, it remains difficult to determine how far any of these samples were representative of the 'true' population of men who have sex with men. The preponderance, relative to the population of the country as a whole, of the more confident and articulate social groups – white, middle-class men in their 20s to 40s – has raised the question of selection bias in all these studies. It may be that we simply failed to recruit the younger and older homosexual, working-class men and men from ethnic minorities.

On the other hand, there is no sound argument for assuming that the population of men who have sex with men has the same socio-demographic profile as the country as a whole. Social and material pressures against homosexuality may be greater or more effective among working class and some ethnic groups while for those who escape such pressures, involvement in the gay community may open up new possibilities for upward social mobility. If this were the case, our sample could well be representative of the 'true' population of homosexual men. Some support for this view comes from comparison with the only British study of sexual behaviour which has been based on a national random sample (Johnson *et al.* 1994). Of over 8000 men aged 16 to 59 who were interviewed, 119 reported having had sex with another man in the previous five years. Among these men, two-thirds were under 35, 95% were white and 68% were middle class.

Talking about sex: Issues of reliability and validity

Just as the accuracy of accounts of sexual behaviour among homosexual men could be affected by how representative the samples were, so they could also be influenced by the validity of the information reported by the respondents. Thus, in designing the research instrument, a range of factors which could potentially distort reports of sexual behaviour had to be addressed, including the desire for social acceptability, misunderstandings of terms or questions and the difficulties of recalling behaviour accurately (Catania *et al.* 1990).

It is commonly believed that the personal and sensitive nature of sexual behaviour make it a difficult area in which to obtain reliable and accurate data. Strong taboos exist against talking about such intimate and private matters and the embarrassment anticipated may make people reluctant to take part in empirical studies. Sexual behaviour is also highly value laden and often endowed with deep emotional significance. Powerful norms define what is 'appropriate' or 'desirable' behaviour among different sectors of the population. Thus, even among those willing to participate in research, the prestige attached to some behaviours and the shame or disapproval attached to others may make it difficult to obtain 'truthful' accounts.

One approach to limiting the effects of social desirability which Kinsey adopted was to use leading questions, along the lines of 'When was the last time you...' (Kinsey *et al.* 1948). By implying the acceptability of such behaviour, this way of phrasing questions makes it easier for the respondent to report them to the interviewer. At the same time, however, leading questions may create pressures in the opposite direction and lead to over-reporting, particularly by the less confident and those anxious to please the interviewer. A more common approach to dealing with the effects of social desirability has been to try to reduce the extent to which the respondent has to reveal himself to the interviewer. In the National Survey of Sexual Attitudes and Lifestyles, for example, the more detailed questions on sexual activities were asked in a booklet which respondents completed by themselves in private and then put into an envelope which they sealed (Johnson *et al.* 1994). Telephone interviews have also been used as a way of increasing the respondents' sense of anonymity and hence their willingness to provide open and honest responses (McQueen 1989).

As in all social research, the validity and reliability of data on sexual behaviour may also be affected by misunderstandings of questions and difficulties in recalling past behaviour (Spencer, Faulkner & Keegan 1988). The sensitivities surrounding sexual behaviour have meant that, in addition to formal 'medical' designations, a wide range of euphemisms, vernacular terms and local street language have developed for talking about sex. Even terms like 'sexual partner' have been shown to have highly variable meanings (Wellings *et al.* 1990). While there is general agreement on the importance of ensuring that terms are clearly defined, however, there is still considerable debate over what terms should be used. Some advocate the use of vernacular terms on the grounds that rapport and understanding are best established when words familiar to the respondents are used. Others advocate the use of more formal terms, arguing that lay terms vary between social groups and that respondents can be embarrassed or offended by the use of street language in interviews.

Differences of views also exist over ways of reducing recall error. One solution adopted by Project Sigma was to reduce to a minimum the period over which behaviour was recalled by asking men to complete diaries of their sexual behaviour on a daily basis (Coxon 1994). This requires a great deal of effort and discipline on the part of the participants, however, which may introduce a marked degree of selection bias in those who complete them. A daily review of sexual behaviour may also become intrusive and begin to alter the very behaviour that is being reported. A more widely adopted solution has therefore been to retain a questionnaire format and to use a variety of strategies to aid recall (Catania *et al.* 1990, Spencer, Faulkner & Keegan 1988, Wellings *et al.* 1990). Building up a framework of significant events or relationships can help respondents gradually reconstruct past behaviour and experience which can then be more accurately described. The time periods selected and the order in which they are asked about can also be important: more recent events are generally recalled more accurately and may themselves provide a basis for working backwards in time. In addition, questions about specific events rather than behaviour 'in general' or 'on average' are more likely to produce accurate information.

Bearing these issues in mind, we designed a structured interview schedule to elicit systematic information on respondents' sexual behaviour and the perceptions, attitudes and social circumstances surrounding it. Respondents were first asked about numbers of sexual partners in the last year, the last five years and over the course of their lifetime. To ensure consistency in responses, a sexual partner was defined as any individual with whom there was physical contact where the intention was orgasm (whether or not this was achieved) for one or both of those involved. Early piloting work had established that a distinction was commonly made between *regular* partners and other partners. The classification of partners as regular or other was left to the respondents themselves, although details of each partner's characteristics and their relationship were also collected.

Descriptions of sexual activities were elicited through a checklist of pre-specified activities. This list was not exhaustive but included all known high risk activities and other common activities. Each activity was designated by its formal term with the more common vernacular terms listed after it. Interviewers used whatever terms the respondent felt most comfortable with, after first establishing the meaning of the term by its formal equivalent. Respondents were asked to 'name' (but not identify) and describe each of their partners in the last month. For each partner, they were asked to think back to what had happened in the previous month and, as the interviewer read out the list of activities, to indicate for each whether or not they had engaged in *that* activity with *that* partner in *that* month. This exercise was then repeated, in less detail, with regard to sexual activities with regular and other partners in the last year.

Using these research instruments, we were able to measure and describe the pattern of risky behaviours among the men in our samples and, on this basis, to estimate the extent of risky behaviours in the population of homosexual men in England. Although we documented levels of high risk sexual behaviour that were substantially lower than the most alarmist evidence produced from early studies of clinic attenders, it was nevertheless clear that sexual behaviour that might expose men to HIV was still common. In the late 1980s, when the first cohort of men were interviewed, the median number of male partners in the previous *year* reported by the respondents was 5, with a range from 0 to several hundred. Three-quarters of the men (76%) reported engaging in penetrative anal sex in the previous year and one-fifth (19%) reported engaging in unprotected penetrative anal sex (i.e. anal intercourse without a condom), the sexual activity with the highest risk of transmitting HIV (Fitzpatrick *et al.* 1990). In the early 1990s, when the second cohort of men were interviewed, the findings were broadly similar (Hart *et al.* 1993). The median number of male sexual partners in the previous year reported by the respondents was again 5, with a similar range from 0 to several hundred. Two-thirds of the men (63%) reported engaging in penetrative anal sex with a *regular* partner in the previous year and 40% reported engaging in penetrative anal sex with a *non-regular* partner. With regard to *unprotected* penetrative anal sex, over a third (38%) reported engaging in it with a regular partner but only 15% with a non-regular partner.

More detailed information was collected on sexual activities with individual partners in the previous *month*. The findings regarding the highest risk activities – receptive (passive) anal intercourse and insertive (active) anal intercourse – are shown in Table 4.1. Once again, there is a striking consistency in the patterns of behaviour reported by the two cohorts of men.

Similar findings for England and Wales were also reported from the work of Project Sigma (SIGMA 1990). As mentioned above, Project Sigma used slightly different methods to collect their data; they also recruited their sample of men from different parts of the country. Although it does not establish the *reliability* or *validity* of the results of either, this similarity of findings using different methods and different samples gives some credence to the findings of both studies. *Direct* evidence about the validity of such essentially private activities is very difficult to obtain (Boulton 1993). Further *indirect* evidence for the validity of the findings, however, comes from comparing rates of 'reciprocal' sexual activities; that is, within each sample, we would expect rates of insertive anal intercourse to correspond to rates of receptive anal intercourse. Table 4.1 shows that this is, in fact, the case in both

Table 4.1   High risk sexual activities in the last month.

Activity	First study		Second study	
	Regular partner	Other partner	Regular partner	Other partner
Receptive (passive) anal intercourse	25%	10%	23%	11%
Receptive (passive) anal intercourse without a condom	16%	5%	19%	5%
Insertive (active) anal intercourse	27%	8%	28%	12%
Insertive (active) anal intercourse without a condom	16%	3%	14%	4%

cohorts, for regular and non-regular partners and for all penetrative anal sex as well as unprotected anal sex (Table 4.1).

A qualitative study of behaviourally bisexual men

In official government statistics of the HIV/AIDS epidemic as well as in virtually all epidemiological and behavioural research, *all* men who have sex with men have traditionally been subsumed within a single category. However, as concern about heterosexual transmission began to grow, attention began to focus on men who had sex with women as well as with men and the previously shadowy category of bisexual men began to be differentiated from exclusively homosexual men. Bisexual men were presented in the media as playing a potentially crucial role in the dynamics of the HIV/AIDS epidemic, acting as a 'bridging group' from the homosexual community where rates of infection were relatively high to the heterosexual population where rates of infection were low. For those concerned with public health, while rejecting the morally dubious concept of a bridging group, it became important to enumerate and describe the behaviour of bisexual men and to develop health education interventions that would be appropriate for this group.

Our quantitative studies of homosexual men proved very useful in this regard, enabling us to report the extent of bisexual behaviour in our samples and to describe patterns of risk behaviour with male and female partners (Fitzpatrick *et al.* 1989). We were also able to describe the characteristics of exclusively homosexual men and of bisexual men and to compare behaviour and changes in behaviour in the two groups. But while such analyses provided the kind of information that epidemi-ologists wanted, other analyses began to point to a greater complexity behind the epidemiological category of 'bisexual' than was generally acknowledged. We found, for example, that there were striking discontinuities between reported sexual attractions, behaviour and self-ascribed identity among the men in our sample. In the first of the Gay Men's Health Studies, over a third of the homosexually active men described some degree of attraction to women but only one in ten described themselves as bisexual and one in nine had had a female partner in the year before interview. Moreover, almost half of those who had had sex with a woman in the previous year did not describe themselves as bisexual while one in twentyfive of those who did not have sex with a woman nevertheless did describe themselves as bisexual (Boulton & Fitzpatrick 1993).

What these findings began to suggest was that bisexuality as a *social* phenomenon was complex, involving at least three distinct components – attractions, behaviour and identity – which did not map on to one another in any simple or straightforward way. But while it raised the complexity of bisexuality as an issue, quantitative analysis of the survey data could provide little insight into how this complexity arose or what it meant in terms of the men's lived experience. Thus, in the midst of conducting the Gay Men's Health Studies, we undertook an additional study to look at the social experience of bisexual men. The aims of this study were to describe, from the point of view of the men themselves, the sexual lifestyles of men who have male and female sexual partners, the way they perceive and understand their lifestyles, and their responses to the risks of HIV infection. Given these aims, the study was designed as a qualitative study where the experience of a small number of men could be explored in depth (Bryman 1988).

Theoretical sampling in a hidden population: looking for bisexual men

Considerable scepticism has been voiced among those involved in public health research, about the value of qualitative research which relies on small, non-random samples which cannot possibly be 'representative' of the population from which they are drawn (Fitzpatrick & Boulton 1996). Such scepticism, however, is based on a misunderstanding of the purpose of qualitative research and the nature of the 'representativeness' of the sample. Qualitative research is concerned not with statistical generalisations but with *conceptual generalisations*; what is important in sampling is not an accurate representation of the phenomenon of interest in its 'true' proportions but the inclusion of the full range and diversity of the phenomenon, so that the concepts and categories developed can be generalised. This is achieved not through random sampling, but through *purposive* or *theoretical* sampling – that is, the careful specification of the factors which might affect variability in the phenomenon of interest, and the recruitment of a sample in a way which ensures that all these factors are adequately represented.

Like most research on bisexual men at the time, our initial quantitative analyses had been based on a sample of men recruited because of their homosexual activity, and for that reason was likely to be biased towards bisexual men who were active on the gay scene. Although we had made an effort to reach beyond the gay community in recruiting men to the Gay Men's Health Studies, bisexual men are particularly difficult to identify and recruit to research. Even more than homosexuality, bisexuality is stigmatised in Western societies and bisexual men may take considerable trouble to hide their behaviour from public view. While bisexual groups have been formed in some large cities, the organised bisexual community is very small and bisexual men generally remain as isolated individuals, invisible within the gay community or the 'general population' and inaccessible for research.

The potential difficulties in recognising and recruiting bisexual men made it particularly important to define in advance the nature of the variability among men we thought important and to target recruitment very carefully so that, as far as possible, the full range of men would be included in the sample. Given the aims of the research, we reasoned that the main factors affecting variability amongst bisexual men were those associated with the circumstances, context or means by which they met their sexual partners. On the basis of our previous research and a wider review of the literature, we defined the main means of meeting partners as including: placing or responding to advertisements for sexual partners; working in the sex industry; living for periods in single sex institutions; membership of social and political organisations for bisexual or gay men; and any other social, leisure or work situation (Gagnon 1989).

Where these means of meeting partners involved an identifiable 'site' and the site was likely to include a significant proportion of men who had men and women sexual partners, it was efficient to recruit from them directly as we had done in the Gay Men's Health Studies. Thus, advertisements were placed in magazines likely to be read by men who were interested in bisexual activities or involved in a bisexual 'scene'. Pubs frequented by male prostitutes and organisations which provided community services for them were approached. The prison and probationary services were also contacted, although no men were recruited to the study through these routes. Two bisexual groups were approached and agreed to publicise the study and arrange interviews. Finally, men were recruited through clubs and pubs in the gay community which were sympathetic to the research.

Where the means of meeting partners did not involve an identifiable 'site' or the site was not likely to include a significant proportion of men who had men and women sexual partners, attempts at direct recruitment would have been too time-consuming and wasteful. Instead, we looked to two other sites which attracted large numbers of sexually active men, a GUM clinic in central London and our own Gay Men's Health Studies. Both these sites had good relationships with a broad range of men and both had additional information about them that would allow us to identify from among them those who met our particular recruitment criteria.

Sixty-six men were recruited to the study but interviews with five could not be used for technical reasons. The final sample of 61 men was similar to that of the Gay Men's Health Studies in terms of its socio-demographic characteristics. Those who took part in the study were generally young (mean age 34, range 19–71), white (57, 95%) and middle class (39, 65%). However, the sampling strategy was successful in recruiting a group of men who were distinctive in terms of significant aspects of their sexual lifestyles. While all had had sex with men in the previous five years, a quarter were or had been married (15, 25%), and as many as a third (19, 32%) were currently living with a female partner. Almost all (56, 93%) described their fantasies and attractions as to some degree both homosexual and heterosexual and two-thirds (39, 65%) described them as more or less *equally* homosexual and heterosexual. Nevertheless, even among this group, when asked how they would describe themselves, only half (34, 56%) used the term bisexual.

Analysing qualitative data: a typology of bisexualities

A particular problem in much qualitative research in public health has been the tendency to conduct only a superficial analysis. Low level, pragmatic categories are developed from responses to open-ended questions and then used to code interviews so the number of responses in each category can be counted (Boulton, Fitzpatrick & Swinburn 1996). However, while simple counts can be helpful in qualitative research, this approach runs the risk of turning the study into a small-scale quantitative study. This is the case when what is considered of interest in reporting the results is the *number* of responses in each category rather than the specification and description of the *category* itself. Where the emphasis in the research is shifted in this way, the work is open to all the criticisms of inadequacy that quantitative researchers are inclined to make.

Our concern in analysing the interviews in our study of bisexual men was to go beyond this level of analysis to develop concepts, categories and typologies which would help us understand bisexuality as a social phenomenon (Strauss & Corbin 1990). While a number of concepts were defined in the context of coding and classifying the transcripts, perhaps the key concept was that of the *sexual biography*. This was defined as the configuration of a man's previous sexual partnerships, *not* in terms of the numbers of partners but rather in terms of the sequence, conjunction and significance of men and women partners. A *typology of bisexuality* was then developed on the basis of the different patterns of sexual biography. This typology in turn provided the main analytic tool for making sense of the men's accounts of other aspects of their behaviour and experience, particularly in relation to how they thought about their sexual identity and the way they managed their relationships with women.

The typology distinguished six different patterns of sexual biography. The first was termed 'transitional' and reflected the process of 'coming out' as gay. Men to whom this term applied had had a history of almost exclusively female partners but at the time of interview had only male partners and intended that in the future this would continue. Such men regarded themselves as gay. A second pattern was termed 'unique' and referred to a sexual biography which, over an extended period of time, was consistently either heterosexual or homosexual with the exception of one partner. Several men described a situation involving drugs or alcohol as inducing this aberrant episode. For a few men, the 'unique' relationship was the physical expression of emotional involvement with one special friend. All of the men to whose biographies the term 'unique' applies viewed themselves as either gay or straight, seeing their identities as unaffected by the aberrant relationship. A third, and less common pattern, was termed 'serial' to reflect a biography in which periods of homosexual and heterosexual activity alternated but did not overlap in time. In general, the small number of men who conformed to this pattern had fewer partners overall than men in other groups. Interestingly, none of the men describing these first three patterns had had both male and female partners in the previous year, and the typology of bisexuality might have looked very different if a narrower time-frame for defining bisexuality had been used (Boulton & Fitzpatrick 1993).

The majority of men in the study showed a pattern of overlapping homosexual and heterosexual partners such as is more commonly conjured up in popular images of bisexuality. Different forms of concurrent bisexuality were also distinguished, however, in terms of the significance attributed to men and women sexual partners. Thus a fourth pattern of bisexuality was termed 'concurrent straight'. Men in this category were involved in relationships with women (usually a wife or long-term female partner) but had male partners at the same time. Among the men in this group, numbers of male partners were usually considerably higher than numbers of female partners and many had just one female partner. While some of these men described themselves as bisexual, many were reluctant to use any term to convey their sexual identity. A fifth pattern, termed 'current gay' is in many ways a mirror image of the fourth pattern. Men described in this way lead open and active lives within the gay community but also had various relationships with women. Among men in this group, approximately equal numbers described themselves as gay or bisexual. An important difference between this and the previous pattern was that the women involved generally were aware of their partner's homosexual activity. A sixth and relatively uncommon pattern was 'concurrent opportunistic'. These men were not in long-term relationships but had sex opportunistically with either men or women. They were generally reluctant to use any term to describe their sexuality.

Qualitative research in the context of quantitative studies

Thus, this small-scale exploratory study was able to provide an understanding of the *social reality* underlying the apparently unproblematic epidemiological category of 'bisexual'. It set out a conceptual framework for distinguishing a typology of bisexuality and provided a fuller description of the lifestyles, and of the perceptions and meanings underpinning them, of a category of men about whom little had previously been known. Within this context, it identified a range of issues which were of concern to particular categories of men and began to define and describe the strategies which they developed to deal with them.

These insights have, in turn, proved valuable to those involved in health promotion, whose tasks in developing interventions have been hampered by traditional stereotypes of bisexual men (as gay men who had married or as young men 'uncertain' of their sexuality) and by rather simplistic notions of a single 'bridging group'. What the evidence of this study makes clear is that bisexual sexual behaviour is considerably more fluid and diverse than such notions would allow. Not only is there substantial diversity, but many men with bisexual sexual biographies do not view themselves as bisexual and do not take any part in social or political activities that concern bisexuality. Nevertheless, what the analysis also demonstrates is that the diversity and variability among bisexual men can be understood in terms of a more manageable typology of bisexualities which identifies a range of contexts and situations which can be appropriately and sensitively targeted by those concerned with health promotion.

Conclusions

As we argued at the beginning of the chapter, sociological research is frequently drawn into research on problems determined by the wider society. It remains for the sociologist to determine how the problem should be addressed and to interpret the evidence obtained. AIDS produced numerous intellectual and scientific challenges for the discipline. The research summarised here instances some key issues that were addressed: on the one hand, how to obtain accurate estimates of behaviour that is difficult to access, and on the other hand, how to contribute to understanding the social experience of that behaviour. Our decisions about approach and methodology were pragmatic and intended to be appropriate to the problem. To estimate high risk sexual behaviour, quantification and accuracy seemed essential. To understand hitherto virtually unresearched issues such as bisexuality, a more exploratory ethnographic style of investigation was chosen. Both approaches are essential to address problems with such enormous implications for society as AIDS has entailed.

Throughout the AIDS epidemic, gay men and health promotion services have endeavoured to use the evidence from social research to design interventions to reduce high risk sexual behaviour. More recently, social research has played a new role in helping to understand and evaluate such interventions. Sociology is therefore continually challenged to contribute to the promotion of public health.

Acknowledgements

The research described in this chapter was funded by the Medical Research Council and the Economic and Social Research Council, and was carried out by Jill Dawson, John McLean, Dilip Lakhani, Rosemary McKechnie and Zoe Schramm Evans. We would like to thank them and the men who took part in the study for their effort and commitment to the work.

References

Boulton, M. (1993) Methodological issues in social research on HIV/AIDS: Recent debates, recent developments. *AIDS*, **7** (Supp. 1), S249–55.
Boulton, M. (ed) (1994) *Challenge and Innovation: Methodological Advances in Sociological Research on HIV/AIDS*. Taylor and Francis, London.
Boulton, M. & Fitzpatrick, R. (1993) The public and personal meanings of

bisexuality in the context of AIDS. In: *The Social and Behavioural Aspects of AIDS* (eds G. Albrecht & R. Zimmerman), pp. 77–100. JAI Press, Chicago.

Boulton, M., Fitzpatrick, R. & Swinburn, C. (1996) Qualitative research in health care: II. A structured review and evaluation of studies. *Journal of Evaluation in Clinical Practice*, **2**, 171–9.

Bryman, A. (1988) *Quantity and Quality in Social Research*. Routledge, London.

Catania, J., Gibson, D., Chitwood, D. & Coates, T. (1990) Methodological problems in AIDS behavioural research: Influences on measurement error and participation bias in studies of sexual behaviour. *Psychological Bulletin*, **108**, 339–62.

Connell, R., Crawford, J., Kippax, S. *et al.* (1989) Facing the epidemic: Changes in the sexual lives of gay and bisexual men in Australia and their implications for AIDS prevention strategies. *Social Problems*, **36**, 384–401.

Coxon, A. (1994) Diaries and sexual behaviour: the use of sexual diaries as method and substance in researching gay men's response to HIV/AIDS. In: *Challenge and Innovation: Methodological Advances in Sociological Research on HIV/AIDS* (ed. M. Boulton), pp. 125–30. Taylor and Francis, London.

Dawson, J., Fitzpatrick, R., Reeves, G., Boulton, M., McLean, J., Hart, G. & Brookes, M. (1994) Awareness of sexual partners' HIV status as an influence upon high risk sexual behaviour among gay men. *AIDS*, **8**, 837–41.

Fitzpatrick, R. & Boulton, M. (1996) Qualitative research in health care: 1. The scope and validity of methods. *Journal of Evaluation in Clinical Practice*, **2**, 123–30.

Fitzpatrick, R., Dawson, J., Boulton, M., McLean, J. & Hart, G. (1991) Social psychological factors that may predict high risk sexual behaviour in gay men. *Health Education Journal*, **50**, 63–6.

Fitzpatrick, R., Hart, G., Boulton, M., McLean, J. & Dawson, J. (1989) Heterosexual sexual behaviour in a sample of homosexually active men. *Genitourinary Medicine*, **65**, 259–62.

Fitzpatrick, R., McLean, J., Dawson, J., Boulton, M. & Hart, G. (1990) Factors affecting condom use in a sample of homosexually active men. *Genitourinary Medicine*, **66**, 346–50.

Gagnon, J. (1989) Disease and desire. *Daedalus*, **118**, 47–78.

Hart, G., Dawson, J., Fitzpatrick, R., Brookes, M., Boulton, M. & McLean, J. (1993) Risk behaviour, anti-HIV and anti-hepatitis B core prevalence in clinic and non-clinic samples of gay men in England, 1991–1992. *AIDS*, **7**, 863–69.

Johnson, A., Wadsworth, J., Wellings, K., Field, J. & Bradshaw, S. (1994) *Sexual Attitudes and Lifestyles*. Blackwell Scientific Publications, Oxford.

Joseph, J., Montgomery, S., Emmons, C. *et al.* (1987) Magnitude and determinants of behavioral risk reduction: Longitudinal analysis of a cohort at risk for AIDS. *Psychology and Health*, **1**, 73–96.

Kinsey, A., Pomeroy, W. & Martin, C. (1948) *Sexual Behaviour in the Human Male*. WB Saunders, Philadelphia.

Lee, R. (1993) *Doing Research on Sensitive Topics*. Sage, London.

Marsh, C. (1979) Problems with surveys: Method or epistemology? *Sociology*, **13**, 293–305.

McLean, J., Boulton, M., Brookes, M., Lakhani, D. *et al.* (1994) Regular partners and risky behaviour: Why do gay men have unprotected intercourse? *AIDS Care*, **6**, 333–43.

McQueen, D. (1989) Comparison of results of personal interview and telephone surveys of behaviour related to risk of AIDS: Advantages of telephone techniques. In: *Health Survey Research Methods* (ed. F. Fowler), pp. 247–52. PHS, US Government Printing Office, Washington DC.

SIGMA (1990) *Longitudinal study of the sexual behaviour of homosexual males under the impact of AIDS*. Final Report to Department of Health.

Spencer, L., Faulkner, A. & Keegan, J. (1988) *Talking about Sex*. SCPR, London.

Strauss, A. & Corbin, J. (1990) *Basics of Qualitative Research*. Sage, London.

Weeks, J. (1981) *Sex, Politics and Society*. Longman, London.

Wellings, K., Field, J., Johnson, A., Wadsworth, J. & Bradshaw, S. (1990) Notes on the design and construction of a national survey of sexual attitudes and lifestyles. In: *Sexual Behaviour and Risks of HIV Infection* (ed. M. Hubert), pp. 105–33. Facultes Universitaires Saint-Louis, Bruxelles.

Part II
Social Divisions, Health and Illness

Chapter 5
Making Sense of Socio-economic Health Inequalities

David Blane, Mel Bartley and George Davey Smith

Introduction

This chapter concentrates on variations in health in relation to socio-
economic position. Other important sources of systematic variation in
health, such as gender, ethnicity, labour market position, region and
age, are considered in passing only. Narrowing the focus in this way
has several advantages. More information is available about socio-economic inequalities in health than about the other sources of variation.
Work on socio-economic inequalities has raised and addressed a number of conceptual and methodological issues which are equally relevant to the other types of variation. The chapter first considers issues
involved in measuring social class, deprivation and health. It then
examines how socio-economic position can affect health. Finally, it
will suggest that a lifecourse perspective provides a useful way of
examining how the life chances of individuals are structured by socio-
economic factors. The chapter assumes a familiarity with basic information on the socio-economic distribution of health (see Primary
sources).

Social class and health: An overview

Social class differences in health have been documented in Britain since
the 1840s. The demonstration that they exist in other industrial countries, in general, happened considerably later. Socio-economic
inequalities in health have been reported recently from a range of
industrial societies as well as from some poorer countries. Comparison
between the size of socio-economic inequalities in health in these

countries is difficult because many different measures, or indicators, of socio-economic position have been used. While the Registrar General's classification of occupational social classes has long been the main measure used in Britain, the data available from other countries are often expressed in terms of education, income or some other indicator. An attempt is currently under way to improve international comparison by using the same socio-economic measure in each country (Kunst & Mackenbach 1994a). The measure chosen as the international standard is the Erikson-Goldthorpe-Portocarrero schema (see below) which has previously been used in international comparative studies of social mobility (Erikson & Goldthorpe 1993).

A major milestone in British health inequalities research was the publication of the Black Report in 1980 (Townsend *et al.* 1988). The report summarised existing knowledge in the area and suggested an influential explanatory framework for investigating the causes of socio-economic variations in health. The four types of explanation of health inequalities which the Black Report proposed are well known:

- artefact
- social selection
- behavioural/cultural
- material/structural.

Considerable scientific progress has been achieved by working within the Black Report's explanatory framework. In particular, artefactual (Davey Smith *et al.* 1994) and social selection (Blane *et al.* 1993) processes are no longer thought to make a major contribution to socio-economic gradients in health. The only remaining doubt concerns what has been called 'indirect health selection' (West 1991). This concept refers to social mobility according to some individual characteristic which is not an aspect of health but which does influence the probability of developing disease in later life; family culture, stability and education have been suggested as candidates. Clearly, there is an interesting scientific kernel to the concept of 'indirect selection' which needs to be retained. This can be achieved by integrating it within the intellectual and research framework which has emerged from the 'post-Black' studies. The new framework takes a life course perspective on the development of disease and its socially unequal distribution, and attempts to understand their emergence in terms of the cross-sectional clustering and longitudinal accumulation of advantage and disadvantage (see Section 'The life course perspective' below).

Measuring socio-economic position

Social class

A range of measures or indicators of socio-economic position have been used in social research. These include the Registrar General's classification of occupational social classes, the Erikson-Goldthorpe-Portocarrero schema, the Cambridge scale, Eric Olin Wright's class scheme, the Deprivation Indices of Townsend, Carstairs, Jarman and the Department of the Environment, as well as single item measures such as income, education, housing tenure and car ownership. In addition, the Office of National Statistics (formerly the Office of Population Censuses and Surveys) has produced a new index of local conditions and has commissioned the development of a new classification of occupationally based social classes which is intended to be in use for the next national census in the year 2000. Most of these measures have been used to explore socio-economic differences in health and the overarching conclusion from this array is reassuringly stable. All are associated with general health and all these associations between health and social position are in the same direction. The most socially advantaged tend to be the healthiest, the least socially advantaged tend to be the least healthy and, in general, there is a step-wise gradient between these extremes, with each incremental change in social position being associated with an inverse incremental change in health.

There are a number of reasons for the existence of so many different measures and indicators of social position. In some cases new measures have been developed because of dissatisfaction with earlier methods. For example, the Registrar General's classification lacks an explicit basis in sociological theory and the perception of this as a serious weakness motivated the creation of more theoretically based and externally validated measures. In other cases measures were developed to take advantage of new data sources; for example, various deprivation indices were created when decennial census small area statistics became available. Finally, new measures can be identified through the exigencies of secondary data analysis. For example, nobody remembers why a question about access to a motor car was first included in the decennial census, but once it had been identified as a powerful predictor of mortality risk its use became routine in analyses of socio-economic inequalities in health. When choosing which measure to use it is helpful to understand their strengths and weaknesses and something of their history and purposes.

The Registrar General's classification has been used for most of the twentieth century and has proved a sensitive discriminator over a wide range of items, including health. This uniquely long time series makes the Registrar General's classification irreplaceable, but certain of its characteristics need to be borne in mind when it is used to study socio-economic differences in health. Each of its social classes is internally extremely heterogeneous and when judged against more internally homogeneous categories, such as civil service employment grades or army ranks, its estimates of the size of class differences in health appear conservative. Second, categorisation of household members according to the occupation of the (male) head of household blinds it to the nature of married women's employment and, by ignoring the difference between single-earner and dual-earner households, makes it a poor indicator of income. Finally, it lacks a theoretical rationale and at varying times has been described as reflecting 'the general social standing of different occupations in the community' or 'the general skill levels of different occupational groups'. Its association with health is consequently compatible with widely different and competing explanations.

Sociologists have long been aware of the atheoretical nature of the Registrar General's classification and several alternative schema and scales have been developed. Goldthorpe has been a leading innovator in this respect; his schema has gone through a number of versions but all have been based on ideas of power in the labour market and the workplace. Goldthorpe's class structure is not a strict hierarchy, but a set of social positions 'identified in terms of relationships within labour markets and production units' (Erikson & Goldthorpe 1993: 29). Central to the schema is the distinction between employers, self-employed and employees. Within the large group of employees, class differentiation is defined according to the nature of the employment contract, which involves issues of job security, career prospects and the degree of trust involved, as reflected in the level of supervision. Subsidiary dimensions are the size of the workplace and its industrial or agricultural nature. An important strength of this schema is that it has been externally validated; the occupations assigned to the schema's various social classes have been shown to be differentiated according to the criteria used in its construction (Evans 1992).

Prandy's work on the Cambridge scale has been similarly innovative. Patterns of social affiliation and friendship and acquaintance choices underpin the scale, which does not envisage social position as a set of social divisions but as a continuum. The scale is an empirical construct derived by factor analysis of survey data concerning affiliative behaviour in Britain. Eric Olin Wright's class scheme is a third alternative to the Registrar General's classification. Wright's class scheme (Wright 1985) is based on relations to the means of production and its creation involved up-dating this concept to current economic conditions and assigning modern occupations to the social classes thus derived.

Few studies so far have used these sociological measures of social class to examine variations in health (Bartley *et al.* 1996). They are nevertheless important in this context for three reasons. First, because each has an explicit theoretical rationale, it will be easier to interpret any health variations which they uncover. Second, in relation to competing explanations of health inequalities, differences between the strength of each measure's association with health will provide guidance as to the relative importance of possible causal mechanisms. As Erikson and Goldthorpe point out (1993: 30–35), occupations which are adjacent on a scale of status or prestige are often found scattered in various sectors of the occupational structure. In principle, therefore, it should be possible to distinguish the relative importance of different dimensions of social position for different health outcomes; for example, whether people with the same level of prestige have different locus of control if they are self-employed or employees. Third, the Office of National Statistics' new social classification will probably have a more explicitly theoretical basis, although hopefully historical continuity will be preserved by ensuring that the new classification can be translated back into the old Registrar General's scheme.

Deprivation

Among the range of alternative measures of socio-economic position are various deprivation indices. Deprivation indices characterise localities in terms of information from the decennial census small area statistics. Each has a somewhat different purpose. The Jarman Underprivileged Area Score (Jarman 1984) was developed to reflect local demand for primary health care services. It uses a number of items, some of which are direct indicators of deprivation and some of which identify population groups at higher than average risk of deprivation. Each item in the score is weighted according to general medical practitioners' judgements about how much it is likely to increase the use of primary care. The Department of the Environment's index of local conditions is used to determine central government's financial contribution to local authorities. It is constructed from small area statistics data plus information from other sources, such as the Family Expenditure Survey and insurance company records. The Carstairs and Townsend indices have been used most often in studies of health inequalities. The Townsend index (Phillimore *et al.* 1994) is constructed from four small area statistics items. The local prevalence of domestic overcrowding and unemployment are used as direct measures of deprivation, housing tenure as a measure of wealth and car access as a measure of income. The Carstairs index (Carstairs & Morris 1991) was developed for use in Scotland, but has important features in common with the Townsend index. Finally, the Office of Population Censuses and Surveys has developed a new classification of areas, containing an innovative element of historical change, which is strongly associated with mortality (Charlton 1996).

Single item measures

Housing tenure and car access can also be used as single item measures of socio-economic position and, when used in this way, have proved strong predictors of mortality risk. Internationally, however, education and income are the more widely used single item measures. Education, whether expressed as the number of years spent in formal education or the level of educational qualifications achieved, tends to be associated with a stepwise inverse gradient in mortality. Most studies using income, whether personal or household annual income or median income of residential locality, have found the same relationship with health.

Summarising the present section, a wide variety of measures of socio-economic position have been found to be related to overall health in a similar manner. It is not simply that the most socially disadvantaged group has worse health than the rest of the population. The complete picture reveals that higher status, income and education are all associated with lower mortality and morbidity in a more or less stepwise gradient. Although the Erikson-Goldthorpe classes, as befits their definition, do not show such an even gradient, overall differences in mortality within this schema, between those with the most advantaged employment positions and those with the least advantaged, are of the same degree as those shown using the other measures.

The stability of this relationship across so many facets of socio-economic position attests to its importance. The next challenge concerns the interpretation of this relationship. How do we explain it? What does it mean? This issue can be illustrated by the numerous possible explanations of the relationship between education and health. Educational success is importantly influenced by the material and cultural resources of the family of origin, so the relationship between education and adult health could be due to the long-term effects of conditions during childhood. Educational success also importantly influences occupation and income during adulthood, so the relationship between education and adult health, alternatively, could be due to the shorter-term effects of conditions during adulthood. Third, some personal characteristic such as intelligence or the ability to defer gratification could independently influence both educational success and receptivity to health promotion advice and, hence, adult health. Again, poor health during childhood could both militate against educational success and lead to impaired health during adulthood.

A similar plethora of competing explanations can be suggested for the relationship between health and each specific measure of socio-economic position. We address these issues in greater detail below. For the moment, however, it is worth noting that one potential advantage of using validated sociological measures of socio-economic position, such as the Cambridge scale or the Erikson-Goldthorpe-Portocarrero schema, is their relative precision about the underlying characteristic being measured and hence their potential to narrow speculation about the causes of their relationship with health.

Measuring health in relation to socio-economic position

Health can be measured in a number of ways and it is important that those used to study socio-economic variations in health are independent of, not contaminated by, socio-economic position. Measures of health vary in the extent to which they meet this criterion.

Mortality is probably the best measure in this respect although it has other limitations, most importantly that the concept of health is not exhausted by the avoidance of premature death. Nevertheless, the recognition that someone is dead and the chances of their death being officially registered are not influenced generally by their socio-economic position. This generalisation is probably more secure in the case of all cause mortality. It is probably relatively safe also in respect of cause-specific mortality, although the officially registered cause of death of members of more socially advantaged families may be biased against stigmatised causes such as suicide, drug overdose or AIDS. Similarly, the most socially disadvantaged may not be subject to such thorough medical examination before death and hence may be more likely to be registered as dying of 'carcinoma; primary site unknown'.

The absence of disease and positive feelings of well-being are more valid measures of health than mortality, but this type of measure is more vulnerable to socio-economic contamination. Many types of self-reported morbidity have been used in studies of health inequalities, for example, symptom checklist scores, rates of utilisation of medical services, the presence of long-standing or limiting long-standing illness and self-assessed general health (Blaxter 1989). In most cases their use can be questioned because to treat them as straightforward measures of physical status ignores the many aspects of illness behaviour which also influence these outcomes. Cultural expectations of health, the nature of one's lay referral system, the quality of medical care available locally, and the demands of everyday life are among the factors which influence an individual's perception of their symptoms and hence their response to questions about self-reported health (Blane *et al.* 1996).

These reservations are relevant in the context of health inequalities because each of these aspects of illness behaviour varies systematically with socio-economic position. The more affluent sections of society have higher expectations of health, more medically informed lay referral systems (Freidson 1970) and access to higher quality medical care. The least affluent sections, in contrast, have more physically demanding everyday lives. As a result all measures of self-reported morbidity are potentially contaminated by socio-economic position. Further, the direction of bias, when these measures are used in studies of health inequalities, is not constant, but will vary with the specific measure used. The more affluent classes, irrespective of any social class differences in health, will tend to report higher rates of symptoms on most measures, for example, questions about asthma (Littlejohns & MacDonald 1993) or osteoarthritis (Hannan *et al.* 1992). Self-reports of limiting long-standing illness, however, will be biased in the opposite direction because symptoms are more likely to be perceived as limiting due to the greater physical demands of everyday working-class life.

Studies of health inequalities have also used structured questionnaires, such as MRC bronchitis, Rose angina and the General Health Questionnaire, and physiological measurements, such as height, weight, spirometry and sphygmomanometry. These measures may appear to avoid socio-economic contamination, but they are not without their own problems. For example, there is some evidence that responses to the General Health Questionnaire are socio-economically biased, when judged against clinical psychiatric examination (Stansfeld & Marmot 1992), and the Rose angina questionnaire produces high rates of positive responses among young women whose cardiovascular health is, in all other respects, excellent (Cook *et al.* 1989). More importantly, perhaps, the use of such measures gains objectivity at the cost of losing the global picture of good or poor overall health. It is possible to be healthy on all these measures (body mass index, lung function, blood pressure, etc.) but to suffer from any of a large number of diseases such as osteoarthritis, diverticulitis and cancer.

The ideal method of measuring health in relation to socio-economic position would combine no socio-economic contamination and an overall assessment of health state. In theory a measure of global health, such as the proportion of each social class which is free of serious disease, could be estimated by using a battery of objective measures, each aimed at one of the most prevalent serious diseases in a particular age group. Whether this is a practical proposition, however, has yet to be demonstrated.

Finally, it is worth noting some of the properties of the terms in which social class differences in health are expressed. Standardised mortality ratios (SMR) reflect a class mortality experience, once its age structure has been taken into account. Years of potential life lost (YPLL) reflect, in addition, the age at which death occurred. Disability-free life expectancy (DFLE) combines data on both mortality and disabling morbidity. The size of the class differences, as judged by the difference between the groups at the top and the bottom of the social hierarchy, appear to widen somewhat in line with the amount of information contained (i.e. SMR<YPLL<DFLE). The index of dissimilarity, the relative index of inequality and the slope index of inequality are methods of expressing the size of social class differences in health which use more information than comparison between the groups at the top and the bottom of the social hierarchy (Kunst & Mackenbach 1994b).

Summarising the present section, the measures of health used in studies of health inequalities vary in their validity, systematic contamination and global nature. Each measure has its own balance of advantages and disadvantages on these criteria. Social class differences in all cause mortality remain the most certain evidence for the existence of socio-economic differences in health. Attempts to study the emergence of these differences, and the fact that health implies something more than the absence of premature death, create the need for additional measures. Each of these has potential shortcomings which should be considered when interpreting the results of their use. In the longer term, new methods need to be developed which combine minimal socio-economic contamination and maximum global accuracy.

Social position and health

There are three main pathways by which social position can affect health. It can encourage behaviours which damage or promote health. It can be associated with psychosocial processes which have an impact on health. Finally, its attendant material circumstances may directly influence health. The effects of each of these pathways are probably additive and may well be interactive. In addition, each pathway can affect the others so that more secure material circumstances, for example, may foster the adoption of health promoting behaviour. Despite their mutual influence, distinguishing between the pathways is useful conceptually and for policy purposes.

Behaviour

Health can be affected by a range of factors which may be thought of as behavioural or cultural. Tobacco smoking, leisure-time physical exercise, dietary preferences and the informed use of medical services are the most frequently cited examples. Each of these behaviours varies with social class (Townsend *et al.* 1988)and consequently they may be the intermediate pathway by which socio-economic position influences health. The potential importance of this pathway is increased by its biological plausibility. Carcinogens in inhaled tobacco smoke predispose towards lung cancer, for example, and dietary saturated fatty acids accelerate atherosclerosis.

Certain reservations are nevertheless worth expressing. The first concerns the extent to which these behaviours are conditioned by material circumstances as opposed to autonomous norms or individual choices. Leisure-time physical exercise may be discouraged by occupations which involve heavy manual labour, dietary preferences may have developed in the context of restricted income and tobacco smoking may be a psycho-pharmacologically effective form of self-medication against the combination of stress and monotony. Second, some behavioural risk factors are not distributed in the expected direction. Mean levels of serum cholesterol concentration and the mean number of units of alcohol consumed per week have often been found to be highest in the healthiest and most advantaged social groups. Third, some studies of health inequalities have been able to control group differences in these health-damaging or health-promoting behaviours. Typically their results show that group differences in behaviour explain some of the inequalities in health, but that clear inequalities remain after behaviour has been taken into account.

Psychosocial

It appears that health can be affected also by psychosocial processes. These have been conceptualised in various ways: the level of environmental stress; the extent to which these stresses are buffered by social support; occupations characterised by high demands and low control or an imbalance between the effort and rewards of work. The main health outcomes in these studies have been coronary heart disease and clinical depression. In addition, psychosocial processes have been suggested as the underlying explanation of the relationship between income distribution and life expectancy (Wilkinson 1996).

There is evidence that the level of these psychosocial factors varies with social class. Disadvantaged socio-economic groups tend to be exposed to higher levels of financial worries and stressful life events and to be characterised by lower levels of buffering social support (Marmot *et al.* 1991). The methods of organising production which are physiologically stressful, such as piece work and production-line work, are largely confined to the manual social classes. Virtually all the occupations classified as combining high demands and low control are working class and effort-reward imbalance at work is likely to be found predominantly among manual occupations (Seigrist *et al.* 1990). Psychosocial factors could therefore be an intermediate pathway between socio-economic position and health.

Biological plausibility is the main reservation concerning the importance of the psychosocial pathway. While it is known that psychological processes can interact with all parts of the body's immunological, endocrine and neurological homeostatic mechanisms (Kaplan 1991, Brunner 1996), unresolved problems remain. In particular, direct links between disease incidence and those homeostatic mechanisms which are most directly affected by psychological stress have often not been demonstrated, and the level of physiological stress required to trigger pathological processes remains unclear. Until such objections can be answered, the biological plausibility of the psychosocial pathway will remain in doubt.

Material

Linking socio-economic position to health via material circumstances is the third possible pathway (Blane *et al.* 1997). Almost by definition, socio-economic position is a, if not the, major determinant of material circumstances. There are exceptions to this generalisation, such as clergymen and penniless aristocrats and manual workers who have won large sums of money through gambling. There is also a grey area on the border between manual and non-manual occupations where non-manual status often attracts lower remuneration than skilled manual work. Nevertheless, in general each incremental change in socio-economic position is associated with a commensurate change in material circumstances, whether these are judged in terms of purchasing power, residential conditions, possessions, hours of work or the hazards associated with that work.

Material circumstances, in turn, can affect health. There is good evidence that exposure to particular occupational hazards can lead to specifically occupational diseases as well as contributing to diseases, such as chronic obstructive airway disease and some cancers, which have a multifactorial aetiology. Material circumstances at work are also associated with the risk of accidents and the chances of unemployment, with its own particular health sequelae. Residential conditions affect health through accident risks – particularly to children and infirm elders – atmospheric pollution levels in the locality – which are relevant to a range of respiratory diseases – and residential damp and moulds which appear to be associated with several disease outcomes. Purchasing power and wealth are not only the major determinants of residential conditions, they also influence the range of foods from which diet can be selected, which in turn affects health outcomes as diverse as the risk of spina bifida during embryonic development, growth and development during childhood, cardiovascular disease risk during adulthood and general debility in old age. Disposable income also influences home heating and ambient indoor temperatures which affect respiratory disease during childhood and the elderly's excess winter mortality.

The main reservation about the material circumstances pathway between socio-economic position and health concerns the lack of evidence that it has a major effect on the most prevalent causes of death in industrialised societies. There is good evidence that material circumstances are important aetiologically in accidents and respiratory diseases which are major causes of death and disability at younger ages. The majority of deaths, however, occur at older ages and are due to coronary heart disease and cancers and, among the very elderly, to a range of poorly understood diseases such as Alzheimer's and Parkinson's. The contribution of material circumstances to these latter causes of death has yet to be clearly established.

One, ground-breaking, study has attempted to disentangle the health effects of autonomous freely chosen behaviours from the health effects of behaviours which are conditioned by their material context. These latter 'indirect' effects of material circumstances were aggregated with 'direct' health effects due to, for example, poor housing and working conditions. The total contribution of material factors (indirect plus direct) to socio-economic differences in health was greater than that of autonomous behaviours (Stronks et al. 1988).

Summarising the present section, three potential pathways can be identified between socio-economic position and health. These are not competing explanations; they work together, probably additively and possibly interactively. Important questions remain about each pathway and a general model is needed which can integrate their effects. This is addressed in the next section.

The life course perspective

The burden of disease in industrialised countries is dominated by chronic disease processes afflicting those in late middle age or older.

Evidence is accumulating that these disease processes have long antecedents. The risk of developing chronic disease in later life has been found to be associated with, for example, intra-uterine development, birth weight and growth during infancy. The meaning of such associations is still being debated, in particular whether they are due to permanent biological damage ('programming') in utero (Barker 1992) or to a continuity of social conditions which sequentially affects maternal health, pregnancy and childhood and adult circumstances (Bartley *et al.* 1994). Nevertheless, this new evidence of long-term influences on adult health has encouraged researchers to think about disease in terms of its development over the whole life course (Kuh & Ben Shlomo 1997). In relation to health inequalities this reconceptualisation has been facilitated by the maturing of important longitudinal data sets, in particular the British birth cohorts born in 1946 (Wadsworth 1991) and 1958 (Power *et al.* 1991). These have allowed researchers to begin to unravel some of the complex processes by which health inequalities are produced.

At its simplest the life course perspective reminds us that the social structure does precisely what the term implies; it structures the life chances of individuals so that advantages or disadvantages tend to cluster cross-sectionally and accumulate longitudinally. This process can affect health through each of the three pathways acting simultaneously. Cross-sectionally, for example, an individual whose behaviours include cigarette smoking and high consumption of saturated fats, is more likely to be exposed to psychosocial hazards such as multiple environmental stresses and employment conditions which combine high effort with relatively low reward; and also to be at greater risk of exposure to occupational hazards, residential damp, local atmospheric pollution and financial constraints on dietary purchases. Conversely, an individual whose behaviours exemplify the medically recommended healthy lifestyle, is more likely to be employed in an occupation which offers autonomy and career prospects; and is less likely to be at risk of exposure to material hazards because of non-manual work, good quality housing, rural or suburban residence and adequate income. In each case the cross-sectional clustering of advantage or disadvantage could affect health simultaneously through all three pathways; damaging health in the former case, promoting it in the latter.

The social structure also organises these processes longitudinally so that advantages or disadvantages accumulate over time. The material and cultural resources of a child's home strongly influence their educational success during childhood and adolescence, which in turn is a major determinant of their labour market position during adulthood, which in turn predisposes towards affluence, or the lack of it, during old age. The health-damaging or health-promoting correlates of each of these phases of the life course can either accelerate or slow the age-related deterioration in any body system. Lung function, for example, deteriorates with age and a number of factors are known to accelerate this process, which becomes manifest as chronic respiratory disease in later life. Among these factors are frequent lower respiratory tract infections during childhood, which are made more likely by exposure to residential damp and atmospheric pollution; cigarette smoking and exposure to occupational fumes and dusts during adulthood; and an inadequately heated home during old age. Conversely, an individual who has spent their life free of these respiratory hazards is likely to maintain good respiratory function well into old age.

One of the strengths of this life course model is its ability to allow for considerable variation in individual life course trajectories. During their life an individual may move from a less to a more advantaged social layer, so reducing the rate at which health damage accumulates. Alternatively, they may move in the opposite direction, in which case health damage is likely to accelerate. The model also allows for an individual to accumulate a unique balance of specific advantages and disadvantages, which may affect the diseases they develop and their precise cause of death, for example coronary heart disease as opposed to cancer, while at the same time structuring this balance so that the chances of dying at any particular age are socially patterned.

Evidence is starting to emerge that the life course perspective is a useful model for examining health differentials. Education during childhood and adolescence, first occupation at labour market entry, occupation in middle age and family assets during later life were each found to make independent and cumulative contribution to mortality risk in the US National Longitudinal Study of Older Men (Mare 1990). Limited education during childhood and adolescence followed by manual work and residence in poor quality housing during adulthood was associated with high mortality risk in a census record linkage study in Norway (Salhi *et al.* 1995). Finally, the West of Scotland Collaborative Study found that male mortality and morbidity risk and physiological status were graded according to accumulated social class position during childhood, at labour market entry and during adulthood. A manual social class position at all three points in the life course was associated with the highest mortality and morbidity risks, the highest mean blood pressure, the shortest mean height and the worst mean lung function. All these measures of health were found to improve in a stepwise fashion as the number of exposures to manual social class positions was reduced; first, a group characterised by a manual social class position at two of these three points in the life course, then, a group characterised by a manual social class position at only one of these three points, and finally mortality and morbidity risks are lowest and the physiological values healthiest in the group which had occupied a manual social class position at none of these three points in the life course (Davey Smith *et al.* 1997).

Summarising this final section, a life course perspective on health inequalities addresses the main burden of disease in industrial societies and offers a model which integrates the development of these chronic diseases with an evolving social structure. The usefulness of the model will depend upon its ability to generate new knowledge. Results from the United States, Norway and Scotland suggest that it has this potential.

Conclusions

Socio-economic variations in health have been reported from every industrial society which has studied the issue. The question of 'whether social class differences in health exist?' has, therefore, been firmly answered. At the same time work within the Black Report's explanatory framework has established which types of explanation do, and do not, make a significant contribution to health inequalities. Research can now concentrate on questions of causation. What causes these variations in health and what are the processes through which they emerge?

These new questions raise issues of measurement which we have considered. Answering these questions also raises conceptual issues. What are the pathways by which social position could affect health and how may these be socially structured in relation to the prevalent chronic diseases? It is perhaps inevitable that this research-oriented chapter should raise more questions than it answers. Nevertheless, the emerging consensus among researchers favours a life course perspective as the most promising way of identifying and answering questions about the causes of health inequalities. Such research will become policy relevant if it can identify 'critical periods' in the life course where social policy intervention might prevent further accumulation of health disadvantage. Variation from country to country in the size of health inequalities suggests the search for policy interventions is a feasible objective. The universality of these inequalities, however, also suggests that there will be structural limits to these reforms.

References

Barker, D.J.P. (1992) *Fetal and Infant Origins of Adult Disease.* British Medical Journal, London.

Bartley, M., Carpenter, L., Dunnell, K. & Fitzpatrick, R. (1996) Measuring inequalities in health: an analysis of mortality patterns using two social classificiations. *Sociology of Health and Illness*, **18**, 455–74.

Bartley, M., Power, C., Blane, D., Davey Smith, G. & Shipley, M. (1994) Birth weight and later socioeconomic disadvantage: evidence from the 1958 British cohort study. *British Medical Journal*, **309**, 1475–8.

Blane, D., Bartley, M. & Davey Smith, G. (1997) Disease aetiology and materialist explanations of socioeconomic mortality differentials. *European Journal of Public Health*, **7**, 385–91.

Blane, D., Davey Smith, G. & Bartley, M. (1993) Social selection: what does it contribute to social class differences in health? *Sociology of Health and Illness*, **15**, 1–15.

Blane, D., Power, C. & Bartley, M. (1996) Illness behaviour and the measurement of class differentials in morbidity. *Journal of the Royal Statistical Society*, **159**, 77–92.

Blaxter, M. (1989) A comparison of measures in inequality in morbidity. In: *Health Inequalities in European Countries* (ed. J. Fox), pp. 63–78. Gower, Aldershot.

Brunner, E. (1996) The social and biological basis of cardiovascular disease in office workers. In: *Health and Social Organisation* (eds D. Blane, E. Brunner & R. Wilkinson), pp. 272–99. Routledge, London.

Carstairs, V. & Morris, R. (1991) *Deprivation and Health in Scotland.* Aberdeen University Press, Aberdeen.

Charlton, J. (1996) Which areas are healthiest? *Population Trends*, **83**, 17–24.

Cook, D.G., Shaper, A.G. & Macfarlane, P.W. (1989) Using the WHO (Rose) angina questionnaire in cardiovascular epidemiology. *International Journal of Epidemiology*, **18**, 607–13.

Davey Smith, G., Blane, D. & Bartley, M. (1994) Explanations for socio-economic differentials in mortality: evidence from Britain and elsewhere. *European Journal of Public Health*, **4**, 131–44.

Davey Smith, G., Hart, C., Blane, D., Gillis, C. & Hawthorne, V. (1997) Lifetime socioeconomic position and mortality: prospective observational study. *British Medical Journal*, **314**, 547–52.

Erikson, R. & Goldthorpe, J.H. (1993) *The Constant Flux.* Clarendon Press, Oxford.

Evans, G. (1992) Testing the validity of the Goldthorpe class schema. *European Sociological Review*, **8**, 211–32.

Freidson, E. (1970) *Profession of Medicine: A study of the Sociology of Applied Knowledge.* Dodd Mead, New York.

Hannan, M.T., Anderson, J.J., Pincus, T. & Felson, D.T. (1992) Educational attainment and osteoarthritis: differential associations with radiographic changes and symptom reporting. *Journal of Clinical Epidemiology*, **45**, 139–47.

Jarman, B. (1984) Underprivileged areas: validation and distribution of scores. *British Medical Journal*, **289**, 1587–92.

Kaplan, H.B. (1991) Social psychology of the immune system: a conceptual framework and a review of the literature. *Social Science and Medicine*, **33**, 909–23.

Kuh, D.J.L. & Ben Shlomo, Y. (eds) (1997) *A Life Course Approach to Chronic Disease Epidemiology*. Oxford University Press, Oxford.

Kunst, A.E. & Mackenbach, J.P. (1994a) International variation in the size of mortality differences associated with occupational status. *International Journal of Epidemiology*, **23**, 742–50.

Kunst, A.E. & Mackenbach, J.P. (1994b) *Measuring Socio-economic Inequalities in Health*. WHO Europe, Copenhagen.

Littlejohns, P. & MacDonald, L.D. (1993) The relationship between severe asthma and social class. *Respiratory Medicine*, **87**, 139–43.

Mare, R.D. (1990) Socio-economic careers and differential mortality among older men in the United States. In: *Measurement and Analysis of Mortality: New Approaches* (eds J. Vallin, S. D'Souza & A. Palloni), pp. 362–87. Clarendon, Oxford.

Phillimore, P., Beattie, A. & Townsend, P. (1994) Widening inequality of health in northern England 1981–91. *British Medical Journal*, **308**, 1125–8.

Salhi, M., Caselli, G., Duchene, J., Egidi, V., Santini, A., Thiltges, E. & Wunsch, G. (1995) Assessing mortality differentials using life histories: a method and applications. In: *Adult Mortality in Developed Countries: From Description to Explanation* (eds A. Lopez, G. Caselli & T. Valkonen), pp. 17–30. Clarendon, Oxford.

Seigrist, J., Peter, R. & Junge, A. (1990) Low status control, high effort at work and ischaemic heart disease: prospective evidence from blue-collar men. *Social Science and Medicine*, **31**, 1127–34.

Stansfeld, S.A. & Marmot, M.G. (1992) Social class and minor psychiatric disorder in British civil servants: a validated screening survey using the General Health Questionnaire. *Psychological Medicine*, **22**, 739–49.

Stronks, K., van den Mheen, D., Looman, C. & Mackenbach, J.P. (1988) Behavioural and structural factors in the explanation of socio-economic inequalities in health: an empirical analysis. *Sociology of Health and Illness*, 18, 653–74.

Townsend, P., Davidson, N. & Whitehead, M. (1988) *Inequalities in Health: The Black Report/The Health Divide*. Penguin, Harmondsworth.

West, P. (1991) Rethinking the health selection explanation for health inequalities. *Social Science and Medicine*, **32**, 373–84.

Wilkinson, R.G. (1996) *Unhealthy Societies: The Afflictions of Inequality*. Routledge, London.

Wright, E.O. (1985) *Classes*. Verso, London.

Primary sources

These articles and books provide access to the datasets but are not definitive or descriptive sources themselves.

Cox, B.D., Huppert, F.A. & Whichelow, M.J. (eds) (1993) *The Health and Lifestyle Survey: Seven Years on.* Dartmouth, Aldershot.

Filakti, H. & Fox, J. (1995) Differences in mortality by housing tenure and car access from the OPCS Longitudinal Study. *Population Trends,* **81**, 27–30.

Marmot, M.G., Davey Smith, G., Stansfeld, S., Patel, C., North, F., Head, J., White, I. Brunner, E. & Feeney, A. (1991) Health inequalities among British civil servants: the Whitehall II study. *Lancet,* **337**, 1387–93.

Office of Population Censuses and Surveys (1993) *Occupational Mortality, Decennial Supplement 1979–1980, 1982–1983.* HMSO, London.

Office of Population Censuses and Surveys (Bridgwood, A. & Savage, D.) (1993) *General Household Survey 1991.* HMSO, London.

Pocock, S.J., Shaper, A.G., Cook, D.G., Phillips, A.N. & Walker, M. (1987) Social class differences in ischaemic heart disease in British men. *Lancet,* **ii**, 197–201 (The British regional heart study).

Power, C., Manor, O. & Fox, J. (1991) *Health and Class: The Early Years.* Chapman & Hall, London. (The national child development study, 1958 birth cohort.)

Wadsworth, M.E.J. (1991) *The Imprint of Time: Childhood, History and Adult Life.* Clarendon, Oxford. (The national survey of health development, 1946 birth cohort.)

Chapter 6
Children, Health and Illness

Allison James

Introduction

The image of a sick child is a potent one. Used in a diversity of advertising campaigns for cough mixture, fizzy drinks and overseas charities the listless child, wide-eyed or tumbled on a bed, evokes a seeming 'natural' sympathy. But whether these images constitute a form of 'disaster pornography' used to elicit political capital (Burman 1994a) or, more prosaically, are simple devices designed to enhance the monetary capital of pharmaceutical and food manufacturing companies, it is clear that their power stems from particular cultural envisionings of the child: positioned as vulnerable, dependent and in need of protection the suffering child calls forth our cash through compassion.

Drawing on a range of sociological and anthropological research, this chapter explores the wider conceptual framework within which these images can be understood. It argues that the idea of the sick child is particularly potent for what it represents is, in fact, a condensed symbol of childhood itself through the intensification of concepts of dependency and vulnerability. Any research into children's health and illness must acknowledge, therefore, its persuasive power. In developing this argument this chapter shows how the socially constructed character of childhood has had very particular consequences for an understanding of children's health and illness. In sum, the effect has been to render children's health and illness as, largely, a problem of and for the state and is therefore primarily an adult problem of family or institutional life. This belated recognition is the outcome of an equally belated realisation of the socially constructed character of childhood. Only relatively recently have children's own perceptions of their own health experiences been seen as making an important and significant contribution to our understanding of children's illness. Only through attributing agency to children has it finally become possible to acknowledge the active role which children can, and perhaps should, take in managing their own health. The chapter considers what is meant by the idea of the 'child' through examining different discourses of childhood; and then goes on to show how these ideas of 'the child' have shaped not only children's experiences of health and illness, but also how these same discourses have shaped researchers' changing approaches to the topic.

Childhood as a social construction

To problematise 'the child' is to acknowledge the ways in which discourses of 'childhood' shape not only attitudes towards the child – and in this instance towards children's health – but also to recognise that these discourses create particular everyday and practical problems for children themselves through offering to them visions of what they are or should be (James 1995). Now usually, but not unproblematically, regarded as the starting point for the new sociological and anthropological approaches to the study of children and childhood, it was Aries' somewhat bold assertion that 'in mediaeval society childhood did not exist' which unleashed a stream of research questioning the nature of childhood and its cultural and historical universality (1962: 125). His thesis was that, although children – as younger members of the species – clearly existed in mediaeval times, the consideration given to them, once weaning was over, was just as people. They were granted neither special nor distinctive status and only gradually, from about the fifteenth century onwards, were children recognised as warranting specific and different attention. The task Aries set himself was to document how that shift in perception occurred and the consequences it has had for modern conceptions of children and childhood.

Focusing on the social and institutional context of childhood, rather than attitudes towards children, Aries was careful to point out that the absence of 'childhood' in earlier times, and thus of the distinctive and separate status of 'child', does not indicate a state of unbridled barbarity. Parental affection and love for children were unequivocally present, he suggests, but what was lacking was an awareness that children might require a different and specific kind of social experience: in mediaeval times, once past infancy, children's needs were understood to be little different from those of adults. Thus, it is the gradual social, political and economic institutionalisation of specifically children's needs which, Aries argued, marks the development of the institution of childhood. In this sense, then, childhood is not a natural phenomenon; rather it is a

particular cultural phrasing of the early part of the life course, historically contingent and subject to change.

Although the precise details of Aries' argument have undergone
serious historical critique and remain contentious (Wilson 1980) the
central thrust of this account was that childhood is a social construction.
Such a view poses a serious challenge to the more conventional
accounts of child development and socialisation offered by developmental psychology (Burman 1994b): if childhood can no longer be
regarded as an unvarying social experience for all children, because
expectations about what 'the child' is vary cross culturally and over time,
then biological development can be said to contextualise children's
experiences. It cannot, unequivocally, be taken to determine them. In
sum, what constitutes childhood in any society becomes, in this view, a
particularised cultural rendering of the biological base of infancy.

Attending to western conceptions of the child, Jenks (1982) notes as
fundamental the twin themes of its particularity, in terms of specific
needs and competencies, and its difference from the adult. Indeed,

> 'the child cannot be imagined except in relation to a conception of the
> adult, but interestingly it becomes impossible to produce a well
> defined sense of the adult without first positing the child.'   (p. 10)

These cultural imaginings about the child have, over time, produced for
contemporary Western children a childhood characterised as 'a period
of lack of responsibility with rights to protection and training but not to
autonomy', and is a view which besets children with the obligation to be
happy (Ennew 1986: 21). It represents a particular mythologising of
childhood through gradually entwining the concept of the child with
ideas of otherness, naturalness, innocence and a vulnerable dependence. This, in turn, has made 'the child' a dominant symbol for other
forms of social and physical dependency (Hockey & James 1993).

The upshot of such a naturalised construction of childhood is that
children's roles as social actors have been, as we shall see, often
obscured and certainly underplayed within sociological accounts. The
emphasis laid upon a developmental approach within western conceptions of childhood has led to depictions of children's social lives being
rendered in terms of children's passivity to socialising acts and their
dependency on adults during the socialisation process. Hampered by the
limitations of this borrowed psychological model little recognition was
given, until recently, to children's own contribution to the form and
process of their social lives (James & Prout 1990). Children were simply
regarded as objects in, rather than subjects of, socialising processes.
However, within the last few years, a growing body of sociological and

anthropological research on childhood is beginning to redress this balance. It is acknowledging children as social actors with their own perspective on the world and is positioning children as people 'engaged in social actions, confronting the world, making sense of it and attempting to change it' (Prout & Christensen 1996). Through these challenges from within the new social study of childhood (James et al 1998) perceptions of children's childhoods are beginning to change.

Child health as a problem of the State

A clear illustration of the ways in which concepts of childhood work to shape and are themselves shaped by ideas of the child, and their practical outcome for children in terms of the provision of health care, can be seen in accounts of the history and development of child health services. In these it is apparent that images of the dependent, vulnerable and passive child combine importantly with what Jenks (1996) describes as the idea of 'the child as futurity'. As he observes, such a perspective is not simply focused on the individual child's biological development and maturation but, more complexly, on the idea of the investment in human capital which children as a population promise. Healthy children will mature into healthy adults. It is this view which Armstrong (1983) documents as emerging as characteristic of early twentieth century discourses of medical knowledge. In tracing the history of paediatrics, he plots its shift from a speciality concerned with the diseases of children to its later role in monitoring the health of the child population as a whole, a development which, Armstrong argues, came about as the result of wider social changes in the relationships between children and adults. As childhood came increasingly to be thought of as distinct from adulthood, so medicine came to think of children's diseases and children's bodies as different from adult ones. One of the most salient of those differences was the potential for future development which the child's body represents. It was a 'futurity' vulnerable to the ravages of disease which needed to be nurtured and protected.

According to Armstrong, in the post-war years attention shifted away from a focus on pathology in childhood to a concern to ensure the present and future health and welfare of 'normal' children through the introduction of panoptical techniques for the surveillance and monitoring of childhood populations, such as longitudinal studies of child health and development. However, the byproduct of such monitoring was, ironically, the discovery – or what Armstrong terms the invention – of new categories of 'pathology' within the child population and the relocation of this pathology outside the physical body of the child in the social body of the family: in poverty, in feckless parenting and in dys-functional families.

Other key players in the constitution of child health as a state problem, in terms of the reproduction of the population, were those more radical educationalists who argued that 'schooling could not proceed effectively if children had poor health' (Mayall 1996: 25). Political activists such as Margaret McMillan made sick children the focus of their attention in the first half of the twentieth century, arguing for the betterment of the lives of working-class children on the grounds of the special and distinctive physiology of children's bodies. It was:

> 'a system of understanding ... structured around the idea of growth and development, it allowed for comparisons to be made between children, and, most important of all as a basis for a social policy on childhood, it rooted mental life in the material body and the material conditions of life. In this way working class children could be seen as having been robbed of natural development, their potential growth lying dormant in their half-starved bodies.'   (Steedman 1992)

In Britain such arguments about the nature of childhood and the needs of children led, though only slowly and grudgingly, to the introduction of school meals in 1939 and to an emphasis on fresh air and exercise as an essential part of the curriculum (Mayall 1996).

That children's ill health is constituted through such childhood dis-courses as a political problem is not, however, simply an historical phenomenon. Nor has the state's unwillingness to take on this respon-sibility lessened. The Black Report of 1980 echoed this imaging of chil-dren as future adult citizens in arguing that child poverty was the root cause of adult ill health. It made recommendations for, among other things, free milk, better child health services and facilities, school meals as a right not a privilege and improvements to public housing (Mayall 1996). However, as Mayall notes, these schemes were rejected as too costly and in the state's refusal to shoulder such responsibilities, child health, became seen, once more, as the private responsibility of families and of mothers in particular.

Children's health as an adult problem

That children's health should be seen as the responsibility of adults, rather than in part their own, is a clear illustration of the manner in which ideas of childhood have worked to shape the social and institu-tional practices of medicine in relation to children. It is indicative, for example, of the traditional and often espoused view that children, not yet mature, must necessarily be incompetent in self care and that, in consequence, it is adults who must stand guard over children's health (but see Mayall 1996, Mayall *et al.* 1997). That in a large part this health care is deemed to take place within families is similarly no simple political expedient. Instead, it is a reflection of the ways in which children have been traditionally positioned. Seen as not only that which constitutes the family through filial relations of dependency, children in their immaturity and 'for their own good' are contained within families and constrained by them (Brannen & O'Brien 1996).

It is therefore unsurprising to discover that, until recently, it has been adults, rather than children, whom social scientists have consulted when exploring children's illness. As in relation to other issues, children's views and perspectives have been largely subsumed within those of 'the family' and, what is more important for our present concerns, presumed to be congruent with it (Qvortrup 1994). A great deal of previous research into children and illness has focused on the effects of childhood illness upon the family rather than upon the child.

One of the classic studies within this long tradition is Vosey's (1975) account of the impact which having a disabled child has on family life. In this she argues that parents of disabled children work towards reconstituting their 'family life' within the paradigmatic ideology of 'normal families':

> 'family life does not appear to be undesirably disrupted by the advent of a disabled child because of the ways in which parents construct their talk about this experience. They maintain a normal respectable appearance because they make situationally appropriate use of the normal family in formulating particular accounts of their activity.'
>
> (1975: 56)

Drawing on the offices of medical practitioners and social workers for the legitimation of their suffering, Vosey shows how parents learn to negotiate their experience of family life through their interactions with others. But in these negotiations it is clear that the disabled child him/herself is not seen as having an active role and, in Vosey's account, children's voices speak volumes by their absence. They are positioned within the family as subject to the skills and practices of their parents, and as objects of their concern. Any contribution by the children themselves in the negotiation of a familial acceptance within the rubric of 'ordinary' families remains unacknowledged, if indeed recognised at all.

Prout (1992a) argues that the twin pillars of development and socialisation shape much of the early research of children in medical sociology and that these are approaches which effectively work to exclude children as active informants about their own illnesses. As noted above, these are the very conceptual frames around which ideas of childhood are constructed, providing for a conceptualisation of children's understanding of health and illness as, necessarily, restricted by the incompetence of their age and stage of development. Thus, early studies of children as patients (e.g. Bloor 1978), though embracing an avowedly interactionist perspective, nonetheless negate children's roles as patients in the clinic setting. Parents and others adults continue to be positioned as the key and authoritative informants. As Prout observes, though children are indeed often silent or excluded in clinic encounters these are 'not apprehended as problems for sociological analysis but are simply taken for granted' (1992a: 131).

Other studies, such as Davis (1982), do recognise the potential of children as social actors , and even as sociological informants, but remain wedded to the traditional view of the child as an incompetent, non-participant. Indeed Davis's study is precisely an account of why children do not participate in clinical encounters and, retreating to a developmental model of the child, he settles on the explanation that children cannot adopt the persona of patient in the clinic because they lack the ability to describe symptoms and to adopt the sick role:

'such claims have to be agreed by others or even forced upon the child, restricting play, access by friends and so on. Again, while the object experiencing the illness is the child, the issue seems to be whether the parents organise the sick role for the child. It is not just assumed.' (1982: 26)

Thus Davis's study, entitled *Children in Clinics* is, in the final analysis, a study of adults' treatment of and opinions about children as patients in clinics. The child remains an object, not a subject, in the encounters between adults.

Other research into children and disability has similarly tended to focus attention on the disability rather than the child, thereby favouring the perception that children's disabilities be seen within particular medical frameworks – the particular needs of children with cerebral palsy, with cancer, with muscular dystrophy. This is again suggestive of an adult bias in such research. The discourses of childhood vulnerability and dependence within which those 'needs' are embedded are frequently the practical, care-taking needs which particular conditions generate for adult carers. Far less common is research work with a more child-centred viewpoint which explores the needs generated by and of the child, rather than the disability. As Philip and Duckworth crisply observe, drawing on Booth's (1978) study of how parents learn about mental handicap in their newborn children, when a child is born with disabilities it is the parents', rather than the child's, expectations and assumptions about children's childhoods which are violated. As it is, from the child's point of view, there may be any number of commonalities in the experience of being an ill or disabled child which are shared across discrete medicalised categories of illness. In contrast, those children who do share the same disability may, depending on their own life circumstances, have widely different social experiences and opportunities.

Philip and Duckworth (1982) argue that what needs to be recognised for children, as well as for adults, is the important distinction to be made between impairment – the loss of function – and handicap/disability – the physical and social consequences of that loss:

> 'many children with diseases, though inevitably impaired, are not disabled or handicapped and many are seriously disabled and handicapped who are only minimally impaired.'   (1982: 10)

Yet despite the urgency of their call for more child-centred research, which could explore the attitudes and opinions of disabled children themselves as Ablon (1990) does for children with dwarfism, only recently is this beginning to be realised within the sociology of medicine. As Alderson (1993) has remarked, even much current recent research continues to see adults, (and especially mothers) rather than children as the clients of health services.

A final indication of the extent to which sociological research has largely positioned children's health as an adult problem is that the weight of previous research has fallen squarely within the field of serious or chronic illness. While conditions such as Down's syndrome, cerebral palsy, visual or aural impairment create serious and special problems for children much of the research work remains focused on the practical, social, economic and emotional difficulties posed for adults who care for such children (Baum *et al.* 1990). While these may indeed be greater and more pressing than those arising from more common childhood illnesses, it is the latter – measles, chicken pox, stomach-aches – which most, if not all, children experience. This also includes those children who have chronic or disabling conditions. Yet we still know relatively little about children's experiences of these illnesses or the ways in which common childhood sickness impacts upon the social worlds of adults and children. The suspicion is that, for adults, such illnesses are minimally disruptive and have therefore sparked off little of the sociological imagination it takes to initiate a research project.

Children's experience of illness

With a few notable exceptions, it is only fairly recently that children's perspectives on health and illness have become a focus of sociological research although this does not mean that research into children's understanding and experience of illness has been lacking. On the contrary, there is a long-standing tradition of research which has explored children's understanding of the body and its functioning within the rubric of a Piagetian model (e.g. Bibace & Walsh 1979). This has largely favoured or been modelled on a developmental psychological approach and uses techniques of testing and experimentation to assess children's understanding. For example, though notable for its early recognition of the importance of the social context in exploring issues of children's health, Campbell's (1975) work on the development of children's concepts of illness remains locked into an explanation based on the staged progression of children's developing comprehension and competence. More generally, such work offers an account of the differences between children's and adults' views in terms of the former's lack of experience and cognitive development when compared to the latter. However, in Bibace and Walsh's study both adults and children make frequent 'magical' statements about their experiences and understandings of illness. As Prout (1992a) wryly observes this rather begs the question about what gloss can be put on the supposed differences between the views of adults and children.

If we are to take seriously the suggestion that children can be regarded as social actors with their own perspective on the social world and with a particular contribution to make, then research into children and illness has to abandon the assumption of differences in children's experiences as being simply a function of age or developmental stage. This is not to say that differences do not occur but to argue that these may be as a result, rather than a cause, of the differences in the social contexts in which children and adults experience health and illness. For example, to what extent do boys' health experiences differ from those of girls ? That they might vary considerably can be glimpsed from Prendergast's (1992) account of girls' experience of menstruation at school, but few other studies make gender differences in children's health a focus. And what difference might membership of different ethnic groups make to children's experiences and their rights in and to health care? Here, too, there is little guidance in the literature, though work in developing countries, where children are trained as health promoters, is offering evidence of children's competence in health care (Save the Children Fund 1995).

One way to begin to explore this is to take up the suggestion of Prout and Christensen that children experience and learn about health and illness 'through their participation in the cultural performance of sickness' (1996: 34). They argue that sickness

> 'can be viewed as a process concept through which different worrisome biological or behavioural signs and changes get a socially recognisable meaning which constitutes them as "symptoms". The result then constitutes the person's sickness in a given culture. This approach implies a focus on how disease (biological pathologies and abnormalities) and illness (personal sensations and experiences) are socialised and the means by which social relations create, form and distribute sickness.'   (p. 35)

Such an emphasis allows us not only to explore specific instances of childhood illness from a child's, rather than an adult's perspective, but, perhaps more importantly in relation to childhood illness, it permits us to see 'fundamental aspects of the social processes that occur between children and adults ... [such as] child–adult hierarchies, relations of power and the distribution of knowledge' (1996: 35). That is to say, it allows us to see not only how the institution of childhood works to shape and pattern children's experiences of illness but how, through a focus on children as social actors, children negotiate the discourses of childhood which they encounter.

We get a glimpse of this potential in Burton's (1975) early and significant breaking of the mould of the more traditional studies of the impact of childhood illness on family life. Her research into families with children who have cystic fibrosis gives some prominence to children's own views on what it is like to have this condition. These narratives are placed alongside those of their parents to give a more rounded depiction of what life is like for families whose children are chronically ill. As do the parents in Vosey's (1975) account, these families endeavour to normalise life for their children, underplaying the difference having a sick child can make. What the children's accounts provide us with, however, is an understanding of how such strategies for masking difference may falter when children step outside the protective confines of the family. As bearers of small, thin bodies it is, for example, when undressing for PE lessons, buying new clothes or in the comparison of body size as part of a measurement exercise in new maths that children keenly feel the potential stigma of their illness through the very public revelation of their bodily difference.

More recently, Bluebond-Langner (1991) has taken this deconstuction of the hegemonic family still further in her study of the well siblings of children with cystic fibrosis. In this account we see how these children take on some of the attributes of what Goffman (1968) calls 'the wise', through sharing secretly in the knowledge about the progress of their siblings' illness. Moreover, as she makes abundantly clear, the extent and accuracy of their knowledge is not conditioned or limited by an age-based competence to know, but related, instead, to the stages in the progression of their siblings' disease. It is an experiential knowledge gained from living in such a family.

In this sensitive and closely documented account Bluebond-Langner builds on the pioneering ethnographic methods she used previously in her now classic study of children with cancer. Remarkable not only for its early emphasis on exploring the social worlds of children, this piece of research offers a detailed account of just how it is that children learn about their illness. She begins from the assumption of children's competence and, in her account of children in hospital, they are revealed as watchful observers and commentators on the process and progress of their own illness. Through noting the changing behaviour of those adults who care for them, learning the meanings of particular hospital routines and coming to understand the significance of certain kinds of medication, the children build up their knowledge of their own prognosis and that of the other children in the ward. They also develop strategies for protecting those adults whom they care for – their parents – from knowing that they know. In this way Bluebond-Langner vividly demonstrates for us children's engagement with and challenge to the ideologies and discourses of childhood which so painfully shape their lives:

'If the staff or the parents avoided the children's rooms too much, the children sensed it was because the adults were uncomfortable about their conditions and "afraid that the subject of prognosis might come up". "No one comes to see me any more. I'm dying and I look bad." "They don't make me get needles no more. Roberta didn't come for two days". Similarly, the children's avoidance of adults, through the various strategies for inhibiting conversation, aroused the staff's suspicions that the children knew, but were not telling. "She knows. She just doesn't want to talk about it". "He yells so I can have an excuse for leaving". As with crying, the children risked being deserted for the action but they also reinforced the adults' belief that the children were normal. Normal children let off steam. They resist passivity. The leukemics' yelling and screaming was seen as fighting, as throwing off passivity, as living and not dying.'　　　(Bluebond-Langner 1978: 207)

Bluebond-Langner's work represents, therefore, an early indication of the power and potential of what later has come to be understood as the patterned cultural performance of childhood sickness (Prout & Christensen 1996).

Such close ethnographic work in which researchers work with children as articulate and knowing subjects is not limited to studies of children with life threatening diseases. Other recent research also takes up the challenge to explore children's own perspectives on health, but engages with the more everyday illnesses of childhood. In Prout's (1992b) study, for example, he explores the ways in which children negotiate the sick role (pace Parsons) with their mothers in accordance with the perceived demands of school-work routines. In the time period prior to the entry tests which would facilitate transition to secondary school, children's absences from school were considerably reduced. Not only were children's claims to sickness discouraged by their parents but children themselves feigned wellness and disguised their symptoms in order to be allowed to go to school or to align the 'end' of a period of sickness with the weekly pattern of school work.

In a similar vein, Christensen's (1993) account of playground accidents underlines the importance of the temporal structuring of children's illness. Noting that teachers (and other adults) often remark on the mismatch between children's complaints about pain or illness and the speed of their recovery, Christensen urges us to consider children's own views. As she remarks, teachers often require demonstration of enduring symptoms (a view stemming from belief in the medical model) before claims to illness by the child are validated (a view emanating from a developmental perspective on children's competence). However, if we focus on the meanings which children themselves attribute to such events, through observing the ways in which accidents are 'performed' by children among their peers, we can see that children's understandings of trauma are differently framed. Children fall over and lie still on the ground, a bodily change occurs and the injured child demands that others: 'Look!' This performance, Christensen suggests, tells us that children are simply requesting that others share in this bodily experience. Thus, when children bring a bruise or cut to an adult's attention they may not necessarily be requesting help or intervention from a teacher because of the severity of the accident; they may just be asking for some acknowledgement of the changed nature of their bodies.

Engaging with this theme of contested readings of children's health and illness behaviour, Mayall's (1996) study follows children across the twin arenas of home and school and shows how children are caught between their different demands. She argues that ideas of children's bodily competence differ between these domains so that children who are ill or who have an accident have to know how to act appropriately in each context:

'at school children have to unlearn what they learn at home. Learning to manage one's own body to suit its needs is valued at home, but that

learning has to give way to having one's body managed to suit the
school timetable ... [and] the value assigned to children's self-care
actions is high at home compared to school.'   (Mayall 1996: 147)

Such differences, according to Mayall, are a reflection of subtle differences in the ways in which childhood discourses are operationalised at
home and at school. At home parents see children as 'constructive
agents within the family' while at school teachers, working with a more
developmental model, see children as 'the objects of their socialisation
and curriculum work' (1996: 82). Children are well aware that school
staff may not offer the same kinds of care as they receive at home.
Children are shown initially taking responsibility for their own illness or
accidents at school rather than substituting their mother's care with that
from another adult: they ' first turned to another child, or a child might
offer help and sometimes accompanied them to an adult for further care'
(Mayall 1996: 198).

   In a study of childhood identities (James 1993) I, too, have focused on
the ordinariness of common childhood illnesses and explored the ways
in which eczema and asthma can pattern a child's social experiences. Of
particular importance was the variability across different social contexts
in how these medical conditions shape the child's social identity as a sick
or well child. The asthmatic child, whose condition is well controlled by
medication may in the classroom be regarded by his/her friends as
normal, but on the running track have this medication condemned as a
means to cheat. The child with eczema, whose clothed body obscures a
dry and scabby eczematic skin, may find in the games lesson that his/her
identity has dramatically shifted. But through careful body management
and attention to the other social skills of childhood membership – the
physical skills of playing football or running fast and those verbal arts of
telling jokes and conversation making – such illnesses may be disregarded by other children and rendered ineffective as stigmatising
markers of difference.

   These latter examples show, then, how children's experiences of illness are subject to alternative, sometimes conflicting, interpretations as
children move between different social domains. They clearly reveal,
therefore, the value of a performative approach to sickness which can
document the precise ways in which children come to learn about and
then make use of the particular local cultural patterns through which
illness is understood and how these combine with discourses of childhood.

   Other contemporary work on children, health and illness explores the
field of health education and raises important questions about how
children get to know what they know about illness as a social and
embodied experience. In a study of young people and cancer Bendelow

and Oakley (1993) demonstrate that children do have significant knowledge about common cancers, though rather less about gender specific cancers such as cervical and testicular. That they gain their knowledge largely from the television and media and from schools suggests the importance of popular culture as a knowledge source and the health education role to be played by schools. However, although the children were aware of the relationship between health and lifestyle, they did not change their behaviour in accordance with this knowledge. As in the adult population, this suggests therefore that the social contexts within which knowledge is received must always be taken into account in judging its effectiveness to change behaviour. In the school health knowledge is embedded in particular structures of authority with which children may be in conflict and thus the role of the school in health education may be reduced (Bendelow & Oakley 1993).

That at an early age children get to know the hierarchies of power through which medicine is practised and enacted is amply demonstrated by Prout and Christensen (1996). They show, for example, that children learn that taking someone's temperature signals the possibility of transition from the state of wellness to that of illness and that the administering of pharmaceuticals registers a further and higher rung on this therapeutic hierarchy. In a later work Christensen (1997) develops this idea to show how children evaluate the seriousness of their own illness through noting the differences in therapeutic techniques offered by their mother and the doctor. Indeed, from the children's point of view, precisely because they are deemed incompetent and their claims to illness may be viewed with suspicion, it is important that they should get to know these rules. It is through competently reading the symbolic practices of their care-takers that children ensure their claims to illness will be endorsed. As Wilkinson (1988) records, even young children of 8 years old are already competent manipulators of such powerful knowledge:

'They described for me the ways in which they might sit in front of an electric fire to make themselves flushed and appear to have an over-warm forehead, eat soap to make themselves sick, or go to the toilet and pretend to have vomited. These special, factors tended to be superimposed on the changes in routine which their parents still emphasised as indicators of illness, such as the child being slow to get up in the morning or having a reduced appetite.'   (1988: 91)

These skills are, of course not confined to children and in my study of childhood identities (James 1993) I explore the ways in which parents, on behalf of their children, use their children's symptoms to exploit the hierarchies of power which sustain medical practice. Although some of the families of children with common childhood conditions such as asthma and eczema worked hard to normalise their child's experiences, in much the same way as Vosey (1975) has described, other families did not. Parents, who felt that their worries had been ignored by medical professionals or that the impact of their child's illness on family life had been trivialised or underplayed, worked to make their children's difference more, rather than less, apparent in order to gain additional help. In this process it was often comments from their own children which were mobilised by parents as weapons in their armoury. However, in so 'believing' in their children's accounts these parents, ironically, risked their own stories being disbelieved by those professionals for whom children's incompetence in and ignorance of the sick role is seen as a 'natural' reflection of their developmental stage.

Conclusions

This chapter has argued that the study of children, health and illness cannot be divorced from an understanding of the ways in which ideas of the child and of childhood are socially constructed. Further, it has suggested that neither can it proceed effectively without recognition of the active part children themselves have in shaping the care that they receive. The question of competence has emerged as central and nowhere does this acquire more poignancy than in debates over children's rights to decision making in relation to illness. Alderson's (1993) discussion of children's consent to surgery has this issue as its central focus. The study explores the ways in which children are encouraged to or dissuaded from agreeing to painful surgical procedures by parents and by doctors. In doing so it examines the different and often conflicting lenses through which children's competence to take decisions over surgery are judged. When agreement to surgery is given by the child the suspicion of coercion may arise; when refused, then the incompetence of children is often assumed. But in different circumstances, the reverse may also be true.

Alderson notes that 'a common argument against warning patients of risk and pain is that they will refuse surgery because of their fears' and that 'children especially, are assumed to be too immature and easily frightened to cope with this information' (1993: 119). However, as she goes on to show, such assumptions about children's competence, derived from particular ideologies of childhood, sit uneasily with contemporary opinions about children's rights. Thus parents and doctors are often divided between respecting children's rights to know and to make decisions for themselves and their childhood rights to protection and dependency which derive from their status as children. At the heart of such dilemmas, then, are questions of competence, of futurity, vulnerability, dependency and protection. In this sense, the issue of consent contests the very nature of childhood itself.

Future research into children's health must also take account of the possibly different childhoods within any population of children and, as in the adult world, of the potential inequalities and diversities of children's own health and illness experiences. As yet, this research has hardly begun.

References

Ablon, J. (1990) Ambiguity and difference: families with dwarf children. *Social Science and Medicine*, **30** (8), 879–87.

Alderson, P. (1993) *Children's Consent to Surgery*. Open University Press, Buckingham.

Aries, P. (1962) *Centuries of Childhood*. Cape, London.

Armstrong, D. (1983) *Political Anatomy of the Body: Medical Knowledge in Britain in the Twentieth Century*. Cambridge University Press, Cambridge.

Baum, J., Dominica, F. & Woodward, R. (eds) (1990) *Listen, my Child has a lot of Living to do: Caring for Children with Life-threatening Conditions*. Oxford University Press, Oxford.

Bendelow, G. & Oakley, A. (1993) *Young People and Cancer*. Social Science Research Unit, London.

Bibace, R. & Walsh, M.E. (1979) Developmental stages in children's conceptions of illness. In: *Health Psychology* (eds G.C. Stone, F. Cohen, N.E. Adler, *et al.*), pp. 285–301. Jossey-Bass, San Francisco.

Bloor, M. (1978) On the routinised nature of work in people processing agencies: the case of the adeno-tonsillectomy assessment in ENT outpatient clinics. In: *Relationships between Doctors and Patients* (ed. A. Davis), pp. 29–47. Saxon House, Farnborough.

Bluebond-Langner, M. (1978) *The Private Worlds of Dying Children*. Princeton University Press, Princeton.

Bluebond-Langner, M. (1991) Living with cystic fibrosis: the well siblings' perspective. *Medical Anthropology Quarterly*, **5**, 133–52.

Booth, T.A. (1978) From normal baby to handicapped child: unravelling the idea of subnormality in families of mentally handicapped children. *Sociology*, **12**, 203–221.

Brannen, J. & O'Brien, M. (eds) (1996) *Children and Families: Research and Policy*. Falmer, London.

Burman, E. (1994a) Innocents abroad: Western fantasies of childhood and the iconography of emergencies. *Disasters*, **18**, 238–54.

Burman, E. (1994b) *Deconstructing Developmental Psychology*. Routledge, London.

Burton, L. (1975) *The Family Life of Sick Children*. Routledge & Kegan Paul, London.

Campbell, J.D. (1975) Illness is a point of view: the development of children's concepts of illness. *Child Development*, **46**, 92–100.

Christensen, P. (1993) The social construction of help among Danish children. *Sociology of Health and Illness*, **15**, 488–502.

Christensen, P. (1997) Difference and similarity: how children are constituted in illness and its treatment. In: *Children and Social Competence: Arenas of Action* (eds I. Hutchby & J. Moran-Ellis). Falmer, London.

Davis, A. (1982) *Children in Clinics*. Tavistock, London.

Ennew, J. (1986) *The Sexual Exploitation of Children*. Polity, Cambridge.

Goffman, E. (1968) *Stigma: Notes on the Management of Spoiled Identity*. Penguin, Harmondsworth.

Hockey, J. & James, A. (1993) *Growing Up and Growing Old*. Sage, London.

James, A. (1993) *Childhood Identities: Self and Social Relationships in the Experience of the Child*. Edinburgh University, Edinburgh.

James, A. (1995) On being a child: the self, the group and the category. In: *Questions of Consciousness* (eds A.P. Cohen & N.J. Rapport), pp. 60–76. Routledge, London.

James, A., Jenks, C. & Prout, A. (1998) *Theorizing Childhood*. Polity Press, Cambridge.

James, A. & Prout, A. (eds) (1990) *Constructing and Reconstructing Childhood*. Falmer, Lewes.

Jenks, C. (1982) Introduction: constituting the child. In: *The Sociology of Childhood* (ed C. Jenks), pp. 9–24. Batsford Academic and Educational, London.

Jenks, C. (1996) The postmodern child. In: *Children and Families: Research and Policy* (eds J. Brannen & M. O'Brien), pp. 13–25. Falmer, London.

Mayall, B. (1996) *Children, Health and the Social Order*. Open University Press, Buckingham.

Mayall, B., Bendelow, G. & Barker, S. (1997) *Children's Health in Primary Schools*. Falmer, London.

Philip, M. & Duckworth, D. (1982) *Children with Disabilities and Their Families*. NFER, London.

Prendergast, S. (1992) *'This is the Time to Grow Up': Girls' Experiences of Menstruation in School*. The Health Promotion Trust, Cambridge.

Prout, A. (1992a) Children and childhood in the sociology of medicine. In: *Studying Childhood and Medicine Use* (eds D.J. Trakas & Santz E.J.), pp. 123–39. Comac workshop project report, Athens.

Prout, A. (1992b) Work, time and sickness in the lives of schoolchildren. In: *Time, Health and Medicine* (ed. R. Frankenberg), pp. 123–38. Sage, London.

Prout, A. & Christensen, P. (1996) Hierarchies, boundaries and symbols: medicine use and the cultural performance of childhood sickness. In: *Children, Medicine and Culture* (eds P. Bush *et al.*), pp. 31–54. Haworth, Birmingham.

Qvortrup, J. (1994) Childhood matters: an introduction. In: *Childhood Matters: Social Theory, Practice and Politics* (eds J. Qvortrup, M. Bardy, C. Sgritta & H. Wintersberger). Avebury, Aldershot.

Save the Children Fund (1995) *Towards a Children's Agenda*. Save the Children Fund, London.

Steedman, C. (1992) Bodies, figures and physiology: Margaret McMillan and the late nineteenth-century remaking of working-class childhood. In: *In the Name of the Child: Health and Welfare 1880–1940* (ed. R. Cooter), pp. 19–44. Routledge, London.

Vosey, M. (1975) *A Constant Burden: The Reconstitution of Family Life*. Routledge & Kegan Paul, London.

Wilkinson, S.R. (1988) *The Child's World of Illness*. Cambridge University, Cambridge.

Wilson, A. (1980) The infancy of the history of childhood: an appraisal of Phillipe Aries. *History and Theory*, **19**, 132–54.

Chapter 7
Health, Illness and the Politics of Gender

Ellen Annandale

Introduction

The social patterning of health and illness by gender is now well-known within the discipline of medical sociology, indeed the finding that 'women are sicker than men' has achieved the status of a virtual truth. The purpose of this chapter is to trace the theoretical origins of this conventional view in the development of second wave feminism, and through this to throw some light on the associations between the nature of feminist theorising and research agendas as they have developed into the 1990s.

The struggle to establish a feminist agenda within sociology was broadly contemporaneous with medical sociology's own attempt to establish a disciplinary project. Both contested the so-called biomedical-model and sought to found a distinct discipline built around the 'social' rather than the 'natural/biological'. Within medical sociology, for example, Freidson stressed that the biological is *overlaid* by the social with the claim that 'while illness as a biophysical state exists indepen-dently of human knowledge and evaluation, illness as a social state is *created and shaped* by human knowledge and evaluation' (1988: 223 [1970] emphasis orig.). An agenda built around the social was also the decided project of feminism as it sought to establish that gender is socially constructed rather than rooted in biology. When translated into the field of health research, feminism's purpose was clear: to separate sex/biology and gender, and in the process to demonstrate that the oppression of women is *socially produced* rather than *biologically given*.

Until very recently there has been a tendency within medical sociology to construe feminism as a monolith and to attribute to it a sense of essential virtue (e.g. for its reflexive and non-exploitative methodologies). Both of these tendencies have rendered it almost impervious to autocritique with the consequence that the sex–gender and male–female distinctions have largely been left unquestioned. This has had the unfortunate consequence of relegating the field of gender and health research to the sidelines of wider debates within feminism at a time when these concerns are central, as is made clear by the absence of any sustained attention to issues of health and illness in most feminist works of the 1990s (even within much sociology of the body).

In this chapter we work towards a reintegration of feminist theories and the sociology of health and illness by attending critically to the ways in which research on gender and health status engages with sex/gender distinctions. The chapter begins by exploring the theoretical project of gendered difference that was established in contrasting ways by liberal and radical feminisms. We will look at the theoretical bases of the conceptual elision of 'men and health' and 'women and sickness' arguing that while this dichotomous viewpoint certainly does have substance, it is to a degree artefactual. Post-modern epistemologies call for a radically decentred approach to gender where diversity is put in the place of feminist approaches which project universalising assumptions on to the experiences of women and men. In the final section it will be suggested that such approaches can be theoretically and politically productive when exploring gender and health status, but also potentially dangerous in their unwitting complicity with recent changes in late capitalism which draw sustenance from plural forms of identity (including those implicating gender), sometimes in ways that are injurious to health.

Establishing a research agenda: radical and liberal feminisms

Figure 7.1 outlines some key parameters of difference between ideal-typical radical and liberal feminist positions as they might relate to health and illness. Although this division and the labels that are attached to each 'position' are bound to do violence to the heterogeneity of feminist theory, each can be seen as broadly representative of a genre of thought that has animated research on gender and health. We begin by looking at liberal feminism.

Second wave liberal feminism promotes an assimilationist agenda, a vision that 'women really are, or given the opportunity could be, just like men in all important respects' (Vogel 1995: 114). Gender, then, should not be allowed to make a difference, something which can be achieved

	Political agenda	Prime determinant of health	Operation of patriarchy	Solution
Radical feminism	oppositionalist	biological (collapses social into biological)	denies women's biological capacity for health	female control of the body
Liberal feminism	assimilationist	social (collapses biological into social)	denies women's access to valued social spheres	female access to valued social roles and statuses

Fig. 7.1 Types of feminism.

by the removal of barriers – for example, legal, educational, occupational – to women's equality. The concept of the subject (male or female) is that of the rational individual, largely unfettered by biological specificity. The distinction between sex (biology/the body) and gender (social/mind) is crucial here: since men have built gender oppression on top of an elision of sex and gender, claiming that women's exclusion from the valued public sphere is consequent upon their biological weakness or reproductive capacities; it is important to demonstrate that this is really arbitrary. 'Mind' is thus privileged over 'body' and the solution to women's oppression lies in 'a programme of re-education, the unlearning of patriarchy's arbitrary and oppressive codes and the re-learning of politically correct and equitable behaviours' (Gatens 1983: 144). Put in oversimplified terms, women can and should enter the public sphere on the same terms as men. This aspiration has been subject to trenchant criticism from other feminists who have argued, following Lorde (1984), that the 'master's tools will never dismantle the master's house'. From this critical perspective, male bias is intrinsic to the institutions that women want to gain access to.

It is contradictory to expect egalitarianism from structures (such as the workplace) which are intrinsically patriarchal, built around the specificity of the male body, and founded upon a separation of the public and the private. The fact that women have a right to be elected to the British parliament (an institution which fails to accommodate to 'family commitments' which are typically the province of women), but are profoundly under-represented within it, despite a significant increase after the 1997 general election, exemplifies this. Arguably, if the separation of public and private continues to be attached to the male–female dualism, then when women demand to be treated identical to men they may actually deepen their subordination since they will be caught, as Gatens (1992: 125) puts it, juggling both their traditional role in the private sphere and their new found 'equality'.

Research on gender and health status from its inception during the 1970s and beyond engages with the liberal feminist problematic in a range of ways. In the first place, it tends to direct attention towards mindful action rather than embodied experience focusing squarely upon *social roles* and their significance for health status. Although the impact of structural functionalism was waning by the 1970s, its legacy was still felt in research terms, particularly in the USA. Parsons' insistence that individual social circumstances and their social actions are derived from social structure rather than based in biology or individual psychology, vivified research on gender and social roles, even though feminists questioned the normative assumptions which underpinned his work. Thus, as Hood-Williams (1996:5) writes, 'the familiar functionalist concepts of "role" and "socialisation" ... had a new feminist vibrancy breathed into them at a time in the history of sociology when many thought they had permanently expired'.

The underlying aim of much research which carries this legacy forward is to demonstrate that women's higher morbidity is not a straightforward product of their biology, but is socially constructed by their occupancy of gender-specific statuses and the enactment of gender-related social roles. For example, Verbrugge (1985) places biology fourth in a rank order of the causes of gender differences in health, behind 'risks acquired from roles, stress, life styles, and long-term preventative practices'; psychosocial factors (i.e. the tendency of women to be more sensitive to symptoms and to report more than men at any 'objective' level of illness); and prior health care (the tentative suggestion that women's greater contact with health services in earlier life may have a long-term protective effect) (1985: 192–3). The public–private divide was uppermost in the research agenda, notably in respect to the value for health of women's involvement in the world of paid work. Research focused particularly upon the 'roles' of paid worker and unpaid worker in the home, as the general conclusion was reached that 'dual roles' are not detrimental to women's well-being. This seemed to confute the criticism that entry to male-defined spheres on men's terms is not in women's advantage, but it pointed perhaps *less* to the advantages of paid work and *more* to the *dis*advantages in relative terms of working full-time in the home (less social support and the lack of a personal wage and the opportunities for self-esteem that they might confer, for example).

However, it became abundantly clear that it was not *all* women who were advantaged or disadvantaged in ways that implicated gender roles. Hence, there is now a growing body of research which draws our attention to the sheer complexity of the relationship between social roles, socio-economic circumstances, gender and health. Taking just the significance of paid work as an example, it has been stressed that any benefits or strains are likely to be influenced by a range of mediating factors, such as: social class; age; marital status; the presence of dependent children; and the form and content of both paid work and work in the home, to name just a few. It is in this context that contemporary researchers have highlighted the practical difficulties of drawing this body of research together to form any clear sense of the relationship between gender and health – particularly given the diversity of samples and measures of health and illness that have been employed – and in which we can raise a more fundamental question mark over the theoretical value of the focus on social roles and statuses in this way.

At the centre of this criticism is the contemporary indictment of the valorising of the social as feminists in general have sought to reflect back critically upon the sex (natural)/gender(social) distinction that has animated research. Barrett, for example, writes in the new introduction to the 1988 edition of *Women's Oppression Today* (orig. 1980) that her book is remorselessly sociological in its treatment of the question of 'sex' and 'gender' insisting that biological differences have no relevance to the social construction of gender. She now argues that considered thought needs to be given to the ways in which the 'biological' is invested with 'social' significance. Gatens (1983: 149) who criticised Barrett for her treatment of sex/gender, argues that 'the view that consciousness is wholly socially constituted and inscribed by means of a passively conditioned socialisation which in turn acts upon a neutral and passive body is untenable.' Put in basic terms, the body can never be neutral, but calls forth particular responses based on its physicality.

The dangers of such a suggestion, of course, lie in the claim of essentialism or attributing a fixed essence to women be this by reference to biological or to other 'natural' characteristics. This, of course, has been a criticism laid most vociferously at the doors of radical feminism in recent years. Indeed, the project of gendered difference which collapses the 'biological into the social' rendering the body mute and privileging minded behaviour within derivatives of liberal feminism, may arguably be seen as matched in intensity by the collapse of the 'social into the biological' within radical feminism through a valorising of the physicality of the oppressed female body. The contrast between the 'assimilationist' project of liberal feminism and the 'oppositionalist' project of radical feminism is summarised by Di Stefano. Radical feminism she writes,

'celebrates the designated and feminised irrational, invoking a strong notion of difference against the gender-neutral pretensions of a rationalist culture that opposes itself to nature, the body, natural contingency, and intuition. This project sees itself as a disloyal opposition and envisions a social order that would better accommodate women in their feminised differences rather than as imperfect copies of Everyman.' (1990: 67)

The research agenda that has developed out of the radical feminist position is well-known: an exploration of women's common experience of oppression consequent upon male control of the body. Some radical feminists such as Daly (1990) appear to valorise the oppressed female body calling for a stripping away of patriarchy's construction of femininity with its correlate of passivity, recognising in its place: pure power. This oppositional framework draws attention towards aspects of health where female and male experience differ, notably reproduction. Radical feminism came under increasing attack during the 1980s for what was seen as its essentialising and universalising agenda, i.e. for assuming that all women have the same needs and that these are rooted in a fundamental difference from men (Grosz 1990). However, a lively debate continues over whether these criticisms are overstated.

A critical assessment

The broad legacy of patriarchy, as well as radical and liberal feminist responses to it has been to construct male and female health in oppositional and universal terms on biological or social grounds, making gendered difference the a priori basis of research. Thus, although not referring to health, Di Stefano (1990: 64) writes that feminism has used the concept of gender to 'simultaneously explain and delegitimize the presumed homology between biological and social sex differences'. But in the process, with its focus on social differences, it has 'undone one version of presumably basic difference, thought to be rooted in nature, and come up with another, albeit more debatably basic than the previous one'. Eisenstein's (1988: 3) feminist criticism of the consequences of an engendered perspective where the 'differences among women are silenced and difference between men and women privileged; the sameness among women is presumed and the similarity between men and women denied,' applies well to research on gender and health. Simply put: from an engendered perspective health and illness (themselves, of course, more accurately viewed as continua of experience) get drawn irrevocably towards gender opposition, constructing men as healthy and women as sick in the process.

The methodological corollary of an engendered perspective is the built-in search for difference in the research methods that we use. There are a number of ways in which the 'truth' that attaches to higher female morbidity may be constructed. The first of these is through the use of data categories such as male/female, in work/out of work which 'impose boundaries that do not reflect unclear distinctions' (Fuchs Epstein 1988: 337). Most telling in this regard, is the propensity of research which looks at gender roles to get trapped within the ideological context of what it is trying to analyse (Carrigan *et al.* 1987) as gender difference is sought from the outset. It happens, perforce, that gendered assumptions can be *built into* the measures of experience that are employed. One blatant example of this is found in a study by Warr & Parry (1982) where marital status and parental status are used as proxy measures for 'occupational involvement' for women. The authors state that although this is not ideal, it is acceptable since: 'our expectation is that the greater proportion of women with children at home are emotionally involved in the parenting role ... and that in general this takes priority for them over paid employment' (1982: 502). In less visibly sexist terms, it is not uncommon for researchers to make assumptions about what facets of this or that social role are relevant for men's health and which for women's health in advance of conducting research. For example, studies of women may stress social support at work, and the possibility of conflict between 'home and work', while research on men's health might attend to physical hazards to health obviating the possibility of looking at the interlacing of 'family and work' for men, and effectively denying the real dangers that women experience in the workplace (which includes the home). Of course, these problems are exacerbated when men- or women-only samples are employed under the assumption that differences are so obvious that data should be analysed separately, thus making it impossible to conduct systematic comparisons.

A second aspect of the social construction of health difference lies in the failure to report findings where similarities by gender are apparent rather than differences. The resilience of this has been highlighted by Macintyre *et al.* (1996). Recognising first of all the assumption of gender difference which is prevalent in the literature, they go on to state that in their own consideration of a range of data, they were 'struck not by the consistency of a female excess in reported ill-health, but by the lack of the predicted female excess, and by the complexity and subtlety of the pattern of gender differences across different measures of health and across the lifecourse' (1966: 617). They report their analyses of two major British studies – the Health and Lifestyles Survey, and the West of Scotland Twenty-07 Study – which permitted them to explore gender and health using broadly comparable measures for a range of age-groups. They find that even though there was a tendency for women to report their health as 'fair' or 'poor' more often than men in both datasets, this was statistically significant only for those aged 18 in the Twenty-07 Study.

In both studies there were no differences in reports of long-standing illness or limiting long-standing illness, and a mixed picture of male/female excess was evident for a range of physical symptoms and conditions. The only area that seemed to corroborate the 'well-known' picture of higher female morbidity was psychological distress. It would appear, then, that within quantitative research on health status there is a strong script of engendered difference as the reporting of null (read gender non-significant) results is generally prohibited. As Kandrack *et al.* (1991: 588) write, sex differences then get 'magnified, the duality of these "differences" is reinforced, and our attention is turned away from the common humanity which men and women share'. Related to this is the tendency to exaggerate differences as researchers 'report the tails of distributional curves and not their centres' (Fuchs Epstein, 1988: 37).

The suggestion that gendered difference leans us toward attaching poor health to women and good health to men implies that we can deconstruct gender duality and reveal a different picture. Any attempts of this kind are bound to be limited by the (probable) failure to report 'non-significant results' in refereed journals; however, insights can be gleaned from official surveys. To illustrate this possibility we can take, first of all, the distribution of cardiovascular disorder. Although heart disease is widely thought to be a 'male problem', coronary heart disease is the leading cause of death for women in many countries, including Great Britain. Crude death rates show that female deaths exceeded males for 'diseases of the circulatory system' to a ratio of 1.08 in 1994. The picture is very complex, but, as we can see in Table 7.1, even though gender differences are small and there is evidence of higher male severity, women experience a higher percentage of cardiovascular disorder than men, at least in overall terms.

Table 7.1 Severity of cardiovascular disorder (all ages).

	Men %	Women %
Heart attack or stroke	5.2	3.0
Angina only	2.0	2.2
High blood pressure or diabetes only	13.3	16.2
Heart murmur, irregular rhythm or other trouble	3.2	4.2
All	23.7	25.6

Source: Derived from *Health Survey for England 1994*, Vol. 1 (DoH, 1996: 3a).

These data seem counterintuitive in suggesting that morbidity and mortality from cardiovascular disease are not the province of men in any straightforward way. However, the disparity with popular conceptions is easily explained. *Age-standardised* death rates for heart disease, which are higher for men than for women, are commonly misinterpreted as suggesting that men are *overwhelmingly* more likely to die of heart disease than women, when in fact what they actually reveal is male deaths at earlier ages, i.e. *premature* mortality. This is not to suggest that premature male mortality is unworthy of attention, but to highlight the point that heart disease is just as significant for individual women (even though it tends to be experienced at later ages). As the proportion of older women in the population grows, the incidence of heart disease will increase. Already in the USA, cardiovascular disease kills proportionately more women than men (Jackson 1994). Yet studies of determinants of heart disease focus on men, and as a consequence a widespread perception among the public is that heart disease is a male problem rather than a female problem.

While heart disease appears to be irrevocably attached to men, general ill health is typically perceived to be a female problem. Table 7.2 provides some data on this, which can be read in alternative ways. There is a degree of indeterminacy in the data – do we 'see' similarities or differences? We could suggest that in the younger age groups (25–34 and 35–44) there are differences (though not statistically significant) in the direction of more *women* reporting better health (itself contrary to the 'usual' expectation of higher female morbidity). However, though small

Table 7.2 Self-reported general health by age and gender.

Health status	25–34	35–44	45–54	55–64	64–74
	\multicolumn{5}{c}{Age % (number)}				
Men					
Very good	48 (259)	50 (228)	48 (193)	47 (156)	37 (100)
Fairly good	49 (265)	46 (210)	44 (177)	36 (120)	49 (132)
Fairly poor	2 (5)	3 (13)	6 (24)	13 (43)	12 (32)
Very poor	1 (5)	1 (5)	2 (9)	5 (16)	2 (5)
Women					
Very good	53 (281)	55 (249)	46 (184)	46 (160)	35 (114)
Fairly good	42 (222)	39 (177)	44 (176)	42 (146)	53 (173)
Fairly poor	4 (21)	5 (22)	8 (33)	9 (31)	9 (29)
Very poor	1 (5)	1 (5)	2 (8)	3 (10)	4 (12)

Source: Derived from *A Survey of the UK Population*, Part 1 (HEA, 1995: 9).

in percentage and numerical terms, in the same age groups it is also women who report more 'fairly poor' health. The usual interpretation would probably be to highlight gender differences, However, valid though this might be, such an interpretation would direct attention away from the high degree of overlap and the significant number of men in fair/bad health and of women in good/very good health.

The intention in presenting the data in Table 7.2 is not to try to 'explain away' difference. Obviously any such conclusion – which is unlikely to be merited anyway – would require a far more thorough presentation. Rather, the data have been presented simply to suggest that things are not as straightforward as they are sometimes assumed to be. These data of course are contemporary snapshots and we would need to consider the very real possibility that differences highlighted in the literature over the years have diminished over time. In this respect, longitudinal data on long-standing illness show that after two decades of higher self-reporting of the simple presence of absence of chronic illness by women, perceptions were the same for men and women in 1994 (women, however, report more *limiting* long-standing illness) (OPCS 1995).

While few medical sociologists would question the claim that the conceptualisations of *health* and *illness* that we use often do violence to the complexity of experience, it is typical to take *gender* as a given and to think of it as a binary opposition (male/female) irrespective of whether it is construed in social or biological terms. Dichotomous thinking which is intrinsic to Western metaphysics, constructs our knowledge and being-in-the-world in oppositional terms. Yet, as has been made clear, notably through the method of deconstruction (Derrida 1982), even though we view the world through difference, all concepts, all identities are referential, known not in their own 'essence' but in terms of difference *to other* things. Feminists have pointed out that binary oppositions are implicitly patriarchal since their 'very structure is privileged by the male/ *non-male* (i.e. female) distinction' (Grosz 1990: 101 my emphasis). Binaristic structures – such as male/female, instrumental/emotional, active/passive etc. – clearly do not define two equal and independent terms. Rather, 'in each pair, the first represents a positive and the second, a negative value, a derived or lacking version of the first' (Grosz 1990: 93). Thus, the patriarchal privilege which attaches to men *depends* on a contrast with women, for privileges – be they in wealth, power, even health – can only be known through what they are *not*, and in the process women become the negative 'other'.

As a fundamental opposition, *gendered* difference underwrites (i.e. supports) other oppositions which attach to it. Thus, the positively valued 'health' attaches to 'male', while the negatively valued 'unhealthy' becomes the province of women. To make this point is not to imply that people do not *experience* illnesses or that they are 'merely' discursive fabrications. Rather, it is to suggest that when the binaristic conceptual attachments which underlie the aphorism of 'female = sickness' and 'male = health' are opened-up (or deconstructed) it is possible to see that things could be otherwise. It is a *methodological* point, then, that lies at the heart of these comments; a suggestion that we reveal that which is unacknowledged as it falls outside the avowed aims of a text, but which exerts a resistance to its logocentric assumptions (i.e. to the given 'truth' that is implied therein). Thus, we can reveal that which is excluded, is important, but cannot be said when binaristic conceptualisations are left unquestioned.

This methodological point also contains a political message. The political project of many radical feminisms – that we can reverse the privilege that inheres in gendered oppositions and 'privilege the dis-privileged' (i.e. women) – will not work, the reason being that it will just shift the *terms* of the problematic, but *not* the problematic *itself.* To raise a question in overly simplistic terms: what would it achieve to 'over focus' on women's positive health? We could argue that it will just oppress all those women who are 'sick', but who by dint of an association of 'women and (good) health' would get neglected in research and policy terms. Of course, the same argument pertains in the current context of patriarchal privilege and health: when men as a collectivity are construed as 'healthy' relatively little is done to protect their health in policy terms, and those who are ill may experience the heavy stigmas of a status that is equated with the feminine/passive. Turned around, while it is of course important to signal the association between women's experience under patriarchy and ill-health, it is contestable whether there is a major political gain to be found in perpetually eliding the two. If health is complicit with illness, or more importantly here since it is conceptually prior, male is complicit with female, then there is the need to recognise their mutual constitution. It is therefore possible to rupture dualisms and to reveal within any text that which it cannot say. Eisenstein (1988: 8), for example, refers to the need to dislodge oppositions and 'recognise the ground in between'. 'Difference', she writes, 'must mean diversity, not homogenous duality, if we are going to rethink the meaning of sex and gender'.

The implications of recognising the potential of such an epistemology are both fairly straightforward and profoundly difficult. In straightforward terms perhaps all that is needed is to be less wedded to engendered assumptions about the experiences of men and women. Certainly it is possible within existing methodologies to be more reflexive about the concepts and variables that we employ. But it is difficult to know how far such a move can go in effectively redressing the problems, hitting as it does straight into the compulsion to bracket experience under various conceptual umbrellas in analysis. Thus, studies of gender inequalities in health are obviously far more sophisticated than to treat women as a homogeneous group, and they therefore build interactions with a range of other social determinants – notably social class – into their models. Yet, taking social class as an example, arguably all this does is redouble the problem given the violence that is done to complex debates on social inequality when 'social class' is conceptualised in terms of mutually exclusive collectivities such as working class/middle class, or the Registrar General's occupational schema (which have always been very insensitive to gender). Evidently, then, there is a limit to how far we can go in building in other factors to enhance our sensitivity to the hetero-geneity of experience, when they equally involve groupings such as marital status categories which force experience into artificial legalistic divisions. And so the examples could continue. It would seem then, that we need to permit gender to take on a more fluid conceptualisation.

With Kate Hunt (Annandale & Hunt 1990) I have been interested to explore ways in which gender aggregates might be deconstructed through conceptualisations that do not rely upon binary constructs. Specifically, we have explored the possibility that the differences in health (i.e. female health as relatively poor and male as relatively good) that are typically interpreted as reflecting a male/female division may mask circumstances that are more fluid. We used the Bem Sex Role Inventory (Bem 1974) which asks people to endorse (on a graded scale) a series of positively defined adjectives or characteristics which are nor-matively judged as stereotypical of men ('masculine') or women ('feminine'). Separate 'masculinity' (high/low) and 'femininity' (high/low) scores were derived for each person in the sample – 35-year-olds living in the central Clydeside conurbation in the West of Scotland in 1987 – which revealed that although, as might be expected, most men had high 'masculinity' and low 'femininity' scores, and vice versa for women, there was also considerable 'movement' such that, for example, 28.6% of men scored low (compared to 71.4% high), and 31.5% of women scored high (compared to 68.5% low) on 'masculinity' (Annandale & Hunt 1990). The results of the analyses were interesting since they suggested that for a range of measures of self-reported health status, gender measured as a male/female dichotomy lost its statistical significance when 'masculinity' and 'femininity' scores were included. It may be possible, then, that the association of gender and health can be freed from its dichotomous referent and attached instead to a more fluid construction of gender: poor health and good health (or, more accurately, gradations between) are not the province of men or women, but of gendered experience which does not attach in any *simple* way to either.

Although there may be some attractions in this type of conclusion, since it would seem to reveal diversity within women and within men and similarities across 'gender as dichotomy' (should we chose to think in those terms), feminists have been very alert to the dangers of such deconstructive moves. Explicitly it has been pointed out that a turn away from 'gender as difference' ignores the various material and ideological bases of inequality and is, therefore, complicit with patriarchy. Following on from this, concerns have been expressed that if gender is not viewed in oppositional terms, then the category 'woman' is deconstructed out of existence and the possibility of collective forms of resistance and emancipation is lost. Many feminists have suggested that a full deconstruction is never possible. Barrett (1991: 165) suggests, perforce, that deconstruction has been very effective as 'an instrument of critique and subversion', but if you *dismantle* opposition, the powers that constructed it get lost in the process. Therefore, the question that must be posed of feminist theory is: can patriarchy as a consequence no longer influence health? In debates that do not discuss health, these concerns have led feminists to suggest that deconstruction is ultimately a 'tool to be used within practical politics, a critical movement that prevents the settling and fixing of foundations and totalities' (Landry & MacLean 1993: 97). Any contemporary deconstruction always takes place *within* a patriarchal social system which established the binary divisions which privilege men. Thus, Eisenstein (1988: 35) suggests that 'we need to work from a position on differences that presumes a radical pluralism while it recognises the power of discourse that establishes (already) engendered unities'.

In the chapter introduction it was suggested that while deconstructive approaches to gender may have some advantages over the liberal and radical feminist traditions which have been at the heart of research on gender and health status, they may also unwittingly enter into complicity with recent changes in late capitalism which are themselves premised upon the more plural forms of identity that post-modern feminism invokes. It is to this issue that we now turn.

Gender and health in late modernity

In contemporary developed economies self-identity is inextricably bound up with the need to posses and consume market-offered goods (Bauman 1987). Since consumption patterns float free from economic production, it is no longer possible, in any straightforward way, to read experience off social or economic group location (e.g. class or gender identities). Thus axes of power cross-cut gender dichotomies in the realm of consumption as men and women are rendered vulnerable to health-related practices that were once much more closely engendered. Although, for example, practices such as cosmetic surgery are still very much the province of women, there is an increasing media message put across to men that appearance is crucial to success. As an article in the *Sunday Times* put it, the message for men is clear 'change your body, change your life. In short, men are acting and feeling like women' (Helmore 1994: 14).

Helmore reports a significant increase in male cosmetic surgery in the USA, drawing in particular an association between ageing and the market place: 'as corporations "downsize" and offer early retirement, men pay to revamp their looks', he writes, 'to stay vital in the market-place and compete with younger colleagues'. Male toiletries/cosmetics are now a £750 million industry in the UK (Tuck 1997). The retort to this, of course, would be that not *all* men are acting in this way. But this would itself underscore the fragmentation/deconstruction of masculinity that has been accented by sociologists of masculinity who have argued that masculinity needs to be viewed not only as privilege, but as wounded and in need of healing (Connell 1995). Carrigan *et al.* (1987: 15), for example, write that concern today is with 'the restrictions, dis-advantages, and general penalties attached to being a man'. Gender is fractured internally, as was noted earlier, not only through the search for profit in new arenas by cultural capital, but though the articulations of theorists of gender themselves as sociologists of masculinity argue that it is *hegemonic* masculinity (also termed hyper-masculinity) – that form of masculinity which at any one point in time is culturally exalted (Connell 1995) – which is argued to be negative for health, rather than masculinity *per se*. Thus writers have drawn attention to an association between hegemonic masculinity, risk-taking, assaults on the body and higher male mortality (Kimmel & Levine 1992, Stillion 1995). This association would seem to be supported by the fact that even though *overall* mor-tality rates improved between 1982 and 1992, there was a slight dete-rioration among men aged between 26 and 38, something which appears to mainly be a result of increased mortality due to AIDS, suicide and violent deaths, deaths typically associated with 'risk-taking.'

The sociology of masculinity has been useful in drawing our attention to the fragmentary nature of masculinity and the existence of hierarchies of intermale dominance, as well as male dominance of women. Taken alongside the opening up of the 'masculine' to women and the 'feminine' to men, in conceptual terms it becomes possible to explore the impacts of *various* 'masculinities' and 'femininities' (as identities and social practices) for men and women upon health. In the research referred to earlier on 'masculinity', 'femininity' and health (Annandale & Hunt 1990) we found that high 'masculinity' was associated with better health on a range of self-reported measures for both men and women, while high 'femininity' scores were associated with poorer health, again for both men and women. Here it is important to note that the measure of 'masculinity' used in the research was explicitly intended to tap positively valued dimensions – for example, 'assertive' rather 'aggressive'; 'ambitious' rather than 'arrogant.' In conceptually similar research, Helgeson (1990) has employed a different measure which allows for both positive 'masculinity' (e.g. 'self-confident') as well as negative 'masculinity' (e.g. 'looks out for self') in a study of gender and coronary heart disease in the USA. In a complex analysis she found, among other things, that negative or traditional 'masculinity' was 'a prescription for the most dangerous components of coronary-prone behaviour' being the best predictor, for men and women, of heart attack severity (1990: 758).

The impacts of the contemporary economy upon gender and health are, of course, mediated through the restructuring of paid work and the household. A recent report by the government's Central Statistical Office concludes that 'the traditional distinction between woman's role of homemaker and the man's role of breadwinner has been eroded' (CSO 1995a: 7). This is linked in the report to a range of complex changes including: the control of fertility; later age of marriage and increased divorce and separation; and changes in labour force participation. It is not possible to document and debate these changes in any detail here. Notable, however, is the increase in 'economically active' women from just over 49% in 1984, to 53% in 1994, with a projected estimate of almost 57% for the year 2006. This contrasts with an overall decline for men from almost 76% in 1984, to almost 73% in 1994 and a projected 70% for 2006 (CSO 1996). These changes pinpoint a restructuring of inequalities. As Graham (1993: 110) explains, 'the increase in women's employment is closely meshed into the growth of flexible working and service-sector employment' as women experience more part-time work, temporary contracts and lower pay. Alongside this, over the last 20 or so years, the proportion of families with dependent children headed by a lone mother almost trebled from 7% in 1971 to 20% in 1993–4 (CSO 1995a).

These changes pose significant questions for the relationship between gender and health which have not yet been fully explored. Put in oversimplified terms: if gender distinctions are being 'eroded' – or more accurately, restructured – in various ways, what implications does this have for health? Trends in mortality can throw some preliminary light on this question. Specifically, there is some suggestion that the marked female advantage in mortality (i.e. women live longer) which has prevailed for most of the twentieth century may be reducing such that there has been a gradual decline in the female advantage until male and female rates reach virtual parity by the early 1990s, and even suggest a reverse trend from 1992 onwards (Annandale 1998).

Although it is far too soon to draw any firm conclusions from these crude data, they are suggestive of one of three trends, i.e. improvements in male death rates, a deterioration or plateauing of women's death rates, or a combination of the both of these. A review of changes in death rates over time suggests that the first explanation may be the most likely. Thus, male death rates show a very gradual, but continuing decline (i.e. improvement), especially from the 1960s onwards, while for women there is much less change over the same period. A consideration of age-specific death rates by gender adds weight and explanatory power to this trend by pointing to a declining mortality advantage among women in middle and late middle age (i.e. 45–55 and 55–64) (Annandale 1998). Thus, although it is certainly still the case that most women live longer than most men today, there is a suggestion of a reversing trend among specific age cohorts. There is a very strong suggestion that this may be linked to cigarette smoking, a health-related behaviour which is closely associated with the commodification of tobacco use and a relaxation of gender proscriptions on smoking which, given the lag between exposure and the incidence of disease (here mostly lung cancer), may be expected to show up in these age groups at the present time. Today in Britain, an almost equal proportion of women and men report that they smoke cigarettes (Graham 1995). As Graham concludes, the situation is such that 'tobacco-related mortality rates are rising among women in the EC, and the rate of increase is now outstripping that recorded among men' (1996: 253). The trend also pertains to the UK specifically where between 1971 and 1992 male deaths from lung cancer nearly halved, while female rates increased by 16% (CSO 1995b).

These data have been presented to give one illustration of the ways in which more 'fluid' or restructured gender identities or gender 'roles' can turn in on themselves in ways that are injurious to health when they are imbricated in the late capitalist economy. Therefore, while the post-modern feminist emphasis upon deconstruction alerts us to the diffi-culties that arise when gender is viewed as dichotomy, there may also be dangers within its *own* position to which we need to be alert.

Conclusions

The purpose of this chapter has been to explore contrasting readings of the association between gender and health status from different feminist theoretical perspectives. Thus we have considered the agendas estab-lished by liberal and radical feminisms; the criticisms that might be posed against them from the broadly post-modern turn within feminism; and the political dangers that might attach to a deconstruction of gender and health within contemporary patriarchal capitalism. The broad failure to appreciate the fragmentation of feminist theory since the 1980s within the sociology of health and illness is, I would argue, indicative of its taken-for-granted nature as it has been co-opted within the sub-discipline. Since now more than ever there is no *one* feminism, it is important to be alert to the theoretical assumptions that underpin research, particularly with respect to the ways in which lynchpin concepts such the sex/gender distinction and patriarchy can be defined and operationalised. Moreover, every theory has its political corollary and because of this various feminist perspectives are never distinterested in practical terms. Failure to appreciate this dilutes and thereby weakens the very significant contribution that the sociology of health and illness can make to the wider feminist agenda and inhibits our ability to move empirical debates forward.

References

Annandale, E. (1998) *The Sociology of Health and Medicine*. Polity Press, Cambridge.

Annandale, E. & Hunt, K. (1990) Masculinity, femininity and sex: an exploration of their relative contribution to explaining gender differences in health. *Sociology of Health & Illness*, **12**, 24–46.

Barrett, M. (1988) *Women's Oppression Today*. Verso, London.

Barrett, M. (1991) *The Politics of Truth*. Polity Press, Cambridge.

Bauman, Z. (1987) *Legislators and Interpreters: On Modernity, Postmodernity and Intellectuals*. Polity Press, Cambridge.

Bem, S. (1974) The measurement of psychological androgeny. *Journal of Consulting and Clinical Psychology*, **42**, 155–62.

CSO (Central Statistical Office) (1995a) *Social Focus on Women*. HMSO, London.

CSO (Central Statistical Office) (1995b) *Social Trends, 1995 Edition*. HMSO, London.

CSO (Central Statistical Office) (1996) *Social Trends, 1996 Edition*. HMSO, London.

Carrigan, T., Connell, B. & Lee, J. (1987) Hard and heavy: toward a new sociology of masculinity. In: *Beyond Patriarchy* (ed. M. Kaufman), pp. 139–92. Oxford University Press, New York.

Connell, R.W. (1995) *Masculinities*. Polity Press, Cambridge.

Daly, M. (1990) *Gyn/Ecology. The Metaphysics of Radical Feminism*. Beacon Press, Boston.

Derrida, J. (1982) *Margins of Philosophy* (trans. Alan Bass). Harvester Press, London.

Di Stefano, C. (1990) Dilemmas of difference: feminism, modernity and post-modernism. In: *Feminism/Postmodernism* (ed. L. Nicholson), pp. 63–82. Routledge, London.

Eisenstein, Z. (1988) *The Female Body and the Law*. University of California Press, London.

Freidson, E. (1988) *Profession of Medicine*. University of Chicago Press, London.

Fuchs Epstein, C. (1988) *Deceptive Distinctions. Sex, Gender and the Social Order*. Yale University Press, London.

Gatens, M. (1983) A critique of the sex/gender distinction. In: *Beyond Marxism* (eds J. Allen and P. Patton), pp. 143–60. Intervention Publishing, Leichhardt.

Gatens, M. (1992) Power, bodies and difference. In: *Destabilising Theory* (eds M. Barrett & A. Phillips), pp. 120–37. Polity Press, Cambridge.

Graham, H. (1993) *Hardship and Health in Women's Lives*. Harvester Wheat-sheaf, London.

Graham, H. (1995) Cigarette smoking: A light on gender and class inequality in Britain? *Journal of Social Policy*, **24**, 509–27.

Graham, H. (1996) Smoking prevalence among women in the European Community 1950–1990. *Social Science and Medicine*, **43** (2), 243–54.

Grosz, E. (1990) Contemporary theories of power and subjectivity. In: *Feminist Knowledge. Critique and Construct* (ed. S. Gunew), pp. 59–120. Routledge, London.

Helgeson, V. (1990) The role of masculinity in a prognostic indicator of heart attack severity. *Sex Roles*, **22**, 755–74.

Helmore, E. (1994) The new cutting edge. *Sunday Times*. 26th June, Section 9, pp. 14–15.

Hood-Williams, J. (1996) Goodbye to sex and gender. *Sociological Review*, **44** (1), 1–16.

Jackson, G. (1994) Coronary artery disease and women. *British Medical Journal*, **309**, 555–6.

Kandrack, M., Grant, J. & Segall, A. (1991) Gender differences in health related behaviour: some unanswered questions. *Social Science and Medicine*, **32** (5), 579–90.

Kimmel, M. & Levine, M. (1992) Men and AIDS. In: *Men's Lives*, 2nd edn (eds M. Kimmel & M. Messner), pp. 318–27. Macmillan, New York.

Landry, D. & MacLean, G. (1993) *Materialist Feminisms*. Blackwell, Oxford.

Lorde, A. (1984) *Sister Outsider*. Crossings Press, New York.

Macintyre, S., Hunt, K. & Sweeting, H. (1996) Gender differences in health: are things as simple as they seem? *Social Science and Medicine*, **32** (4), 395–402.

OPCS (Office of Population and Censuses) (1995) *Living in Britain. Results from the 1994 General Household Survey*. HMSO, London.

Stillion, J. (1995) Premature death among males. In: *Health and Illness. Gender, Power and the Body* (eds G. Sabo & D.F. Gordon), pp. 46–67. Sage, London.

Tuck, A. (1977) When is a moisturiser a 'face protector'? *Independent on Sunday*, July 20th.

Verbrugge, L. (1985) Gender and health: an update on the evidence. *Journal of Health and Social Behavior*, **26** (September), 156–82.

Vogel, L. (1995) *Woman Questions. Essays for a Materialist Feminism.* Pluto Press, London.

Warr, P. & Parry, G. (1982) Paid employment and women's psychological well-being. *Psychological Bulletin*, **91**, 498–516.

Chapter 8
Health and Illness in Later Life

Sara Arber and Jay Ginn

Introduction

Why is there a chapter concerned with health and illness in later life in this volume? In what ways are issues associated with health, chronic illness or disability any different in later life from other times of the life course? This chapter will consider some of the ways in which the 'traditional fare' of the sociology of health and illness might differ when the subjects of study are older people. After considering the meanings of age, we look at ageism in society and in health care and go on to consider patterns of inequality in old age. The chapter concludes by discussing the policy context of ageing in contemporary Britain.

The changing life course

We first illustrate the changing nature of later life across time, as well as gender differences in ageing, by reference to Shakespeare's familiar characterisation in *As You Like It*, and a recent portrayal by Shirley Meredeen (1995). Shakespeare's life course focuses on men's achievement in the public sphere as 'the soldier' and 'the justice'. There is no mention of the private sphere of home and family, apart from conquests as 'the lover'. Later life (in the sixth age) represents loss of public roles and of a strong masculine body – 'his shrunk shank; and his big manly voice turning again towards childish treble', and the final age portrays loss of bodily capacity and function – 'Sans teeth, sans eyes, sans taste, sans everything'. Women's life course is invisible in Shakespeare's characterisation.

Shirley Meredeen (1995), writing in her sixties, portrays a very different life course, with greater continuity between stages, illustrating women's roles both in the family and in paid work – 'the working mother rushing from job to home, from shop to parent's evening'. It gives a much more positive image of later life, providing new opportunities, choice and autonomy – 'the wise crone ... knowing her time has come for fun', and finally 'Last scene of all, in disgraceful serenity, having shed responsibilities for others, having done her duty many times'. It reminds us that older people enter later life as a product of their earlier life course, in terms of family roles and social relationships.

Cohorts enter later life with differing expectations and attitudes which have been formed by the extant values and experiences of their early adult years. Older people today grew up before the 1930s, prior to the introduction of the welfare state and are likely to differ from people entering later life in the twenty-first century. Meredeen's 'seven ages' concludes '*avec* her own teeth, *avec* bespectacled eyes...' illustrating the differences between two historical periods arising from advances in biomedicine. Shakespeare's 'sans teeth, sans eyes, sans taste', should no longer be a problem for most older people. It draws attention to the importance of adequate optician and dentistry services for older people, as well as hip replacements and aids and adaptations. One could argue that both characterisations omit the final stage of what Laslett (1989) calls 'The Fourth Age' of 'decrepitude' and Featherstone and Hepworth (1989) refer to as 'deep old age'. But this last stage of physical or mental incapacity is not universally experienced and at any one time applies to only a tiny fraction of older people.

A major omission from both portrayals is a sense of the diversity of ageing; gender, class and race differentiate people's life courses, colouring their experience of later life, influencing their attitudes, roles and material circumstances. Different marital, fertility and employment histories add further diversity, but the starkness of such differences is likely to vary between historical periods and across societies. An appreciation of the influence of earlier stages of the life course helps in understanding the health and illness of older people.

The meanings of age

One of the difficulties in discussing health and illness among older people is the lack of conceptual refinement of the term 'age'. This contrasts with the distinction between 'sex' and 'gender', which has become accepted within sociology over the last 20 years. Often no clear distinction is made among the following meanings of age.

- *Chronological age* refers to the individual's age in years. This is the criterion most often used in making judgements about medical treatment, and is enshrined in legal restrictions and privileges. In medicine it is usually assumed to be closely identified with the other meanings of age.
- *Physiological age* refers to the ageing process. It is a medically constructed concept associated with the ageing body. With ageing, physiological changes occur in terms of the composition of bones, the process of degeneration of body tissue and functional impairment, but these changes cannot simply be 'read off' from chronological age. For example, the level of functional impairment of women and men aged 65–69 who were previously in manual jobs is poorer than that of upper middle class people who are 5 years older (Arber & Ginn 1993). Thus physiological age is socially structured.
- *Social age* is socially constructed and profoundly gendered. It has several interrelated meanings: (i) The individual's subjective perception of their age. Older people often say they feel the same as they did when they were much younger, but the physiological ageing process means that their physical image has changed. Featherstone and Hepworth (1991) talk of the 'mask of ageing', arguing that the essential identity of the person is concealed beneath the image of an older person. (ii) Age norms about appropriate behaviours for someone perceived to be of a certain chronological (or physiological) age. (iii) The age the individual is accorded by others, which is influenced by their appearance and behaviour.

A 'double standard of ageing' operates, whereby women, more than men, are judged in terms of the degree to which they maintain a youthful and sexually attractive appearance (Arber & Ginn 1995). Older women are expected to ward off the signs of ageing, particularly greying hair and wrinkles. Medical procedures and products may be increasingly used in an attempt to retain a youthful image, especially the use of so-called 'cosmetic' surgery in the USA. This growing area of private health expenditure may have severe iatrogenic consequences, which, because of the gender bias in usage, will affect women more than men. However, the same concern with appearance may lead older women to take more care than men to eat a healthy diet and maintain fitness. Although responses to the effects of ageing on appearance are likely to depend on earlier lifestyle and on financial resources.

Later life has generally been demarcated by retirement, state pension age or a particular chronological age, although none of these necessarily coincides with health status. Retirement usually represents a greater discontinuity for men than for women, who often continue in some of their family roles. Exit from paid employment is less closely linked to serious health decline than in the past. The late twentieth century has brought an unprecedented conjunction of two opposing trends in Western societies – decreasing age of exit from the labour force and increasing longevity. In Britain, half of men and women are no longer in paid work by age 61 and 57 respectively. The expectation of life at age 60 is shown in Table 8.1, demonstrating that the period after labour force exit for most men is nearly 20 years and for many women spans over a quarter of a century.

Table 8.1   Changes in expectation of life, 1961–1994, men and women, England and Wales.

Expectation of Life	1961	1981	1994
At Birth			
Men	68.1	71.0	74.2
Women	74.0	77.0	79.4
Sex differential	5.9 years	6.0 years	5.2 years
At age 60			
Men	15.1	16.4	18.3
Women	19.1	20.9	22.4
Sex differential	4.0 years	4.5 years	4.1 years
At age 80			
Men	5.2	5.8	6.6
Women	6.4	7.5	8.5
Sex differential	1.2 years	1.7 years	1.9 years

Source: OPCS (1996) Population Trends 86, Table 12, HMSO, London.

The state pension age, which is 65 for men and 60 for women, gradually increasing to 65 for women from 2010 to 2020, is similarly unhelpful as a marker of later life. Although chronological age is associated with increased risk of suffering from mortality, ill health or functional disability, this association with age can blind us to the diversity in health experience within any particular age group. Differences within age groups, for example according to gender or class, may be more important than differences between age groups. There is no specific age at which ill health increases in a stepped or discontinuous way.

Apart from the greater probability of ill health in later life, should sociologists of health consider older people differently, compared with people in their thirties or fifties? In many cases similar issues apply, for example, in terms of lay ideas about health and illness. Class and cultural resources may be more important than chronological age in influencing how older people experience illness and what factors lead them to seek health care or engage in health promoting behaviour. However, there are also specific differences for older people, associated with:

- normative expectations and reference groups
- ageism in society
- ageism in the NHS
- material resources, and
- the availability of family carers.

These differences are interconnected and are specific to our society and each historical epoch. Underlying these differences are gender roles and relationships which take on unique features in later life, and differentiate it from other stages of the life course. We turn to consider these ways in which the experience of health and illness is likely to differ in later life compared with earlier stages of the life course.

Chronic illness and disability 'in time' and 'out of time'

There have been many important and influential studies of chronic illness, which have advanced our knowledge of the adverse material, social and psychological effects of chronic illness and disability, as well as strategies of coping and accommodating to ill health. Most of these studies have been conducted on adults below age 65, yet the vast majority of people with chronic illness or disability are above this age. The sociology and politics of disability have been prominent concerns in recent years and have included feminist writing. However, this body of influential literature has primarily reflected the concerns of disabled adults of working age, rather than the majority of disabled people.

A paradox is that in areas of the sociology of health and illness which are important to older people, such as research on chronic illness and disability, the voices and concerns of older people have been eerily absent (Arber & Ginn 1995). This seeming paradox may be explicable in terms of conceptions of normality and abnormality. For those of working age, chronic illness or disability is 'out of time', seen as abnormal and problematic at a societal level, because of inability or reduced capacity to perform paid work and thus contribute to the formal economy; and at a personal level, by interfering with their expected life trajectory, in terms of family formation, social roles and activities. We suggest chronic ill health in older people has not been a primary area of sociological inquiry because it is 'in time' and considered normal, even though problematic in creating a burden on informal carers and on taxpayers who fund health and residential care.

It is surprising, given the richness of work by feminist medical sociologists, that there has been so little work on older women's health. Indeed, feminist sociologists have contributed to the pathologisation of older women; countless studies of caring have examined the 'burdens' faced by younger and mid-life women in providing informal care for their ageing parents, focusing on how caring has constrained women's opportunities for paid employment and other activities (cf. Lewis & Meredith 1988). Since the majority of older people in need of care are women, such studies have in effect objectified older women as the 'problem', the 'burden' to be cared for, the 'other'.

Demographic change and ageism

A key issue is whether and how ageism – socially created disadvantages or negative attitudes associated with age (Bytheway 1995) – affects older people's experience of health and illness. Societal attitudes towards older people have varied historically and among countries. Increasingly since the nineteenth century older people have been seen as economically and socially redundant, as cessation of paid work (often without choice), has occurred at ever-earlier ages. Increased life expectancy, combined with declining fertility, has transformed the age structure of Western societies from a pyramid to an uneven pillar. Between 1961 and 1994, life expectancy at birth increased from 68 to 74 for men and from 74 to 79 for women (Table 8.1), while age-specific mortality rates have shown a corresponding decline over time, especially for older men. However, the rise in longevity, instead of being celebrated as a major social achievement is often seen, through the lens of ageism, as a problem for society.

Within official discourse on caring all elderly people are seen as potentially in need of care. For example, the General Household Survey identifies carers as anyone who 'looks after (or helps) someone who is sick, handicapped or elderly' (Green 1988). This linking of chronological age with a need for care fuels ageist images of older people as a burden. It renders invisible the services, care and unpaid work they provide in the extended family and to friends and neighbours, as well as their role in voluntary organisations and community activities.

Ageism is most evident in media reports of the 'Grey time bomb' or the 'rising tide' in which the growth of the older population is portrayed as creating an increasingly unaffordable burden on society, through the cost of public pensions and health care. This alarmism, or moral panic, has become part of the everyday repertoire of the media and politicians. Alarmism about the growth in the older population has been even more vociferous in the USA, where the term 'apocalyptic demography' is used. Concerns about 'intergenerational inequity' have become prominent in the USA with older people seen as wealthy and privileged in their receipt of health care, benefiting at the expense of other deserving groups, especially families with children. Minkler (1991) characterises this 'canes (walking sticks) vs kids' argument as a false opposition, pointing out that there is seldom any debate in the media concerning competition between the military budget and older people for public funds. However, 'where a hypothetical 'guns vs canes' trade-off is proposed, the American public overwhelmingly supports the latter' (Minkler 1991: 76).

The projected increase in the proportion of older people in Britain is modest relative to past change. For example, the proportion of the population aged over 65 grew from 13% in 1971 to 16% in 1981, and remained stable at this level until 1995. It is projected to fall to 15% by 2001, and rise to 17% by 2011 (CSO 1996). Although the proportion of people aged over 85 has doubled from 1971 to 1995, it represents a tiny fraction of the population.

Most important, the health care needs and costs for older people cannot simply be read off from their numbers, for several reasons. First, the health status of older people is better now than in the past. An extensive debate has raged in the USA for the last 15 years about whether longer life is associated with an increased period of incapacity and dependency in the final years (Verbrugge 1989) or longer active life with a shorter period of ill health or disability – 'compression of morbidity' – preceding death (Fries 1989). A range of methodologically sophisticated population-based research studies were funded to answer this question. There is now incontrovertible US evidence that older people have lower levels of disability and fewer chronic disabling conditions now than in the past. Manton and his colleagues (1995) used longitudinal data from 1982 to 1989 to document the age–sex standardised decline in disabling conditions, especially in heart and circulatory conditions. The probability that a person age 85 or older remained free of disabilities increased by nearly 30% over this 7-year period. Preliminary findings from their 1994 follow-up suggest further drops in disability. It is remarkable that there has been so little attempt in Britain to answer this question, especially given the spate of rhetoric and alarmist panic about the growth in the older population. The Medical Research Council (MRC) concluded 'It is a matter of profound concern that it is currently not possible to determine whether the health status of the older population has improved, deteriorated or remained the same during the past decades of mortality decline' (1994: 26).

Second, health care costs are not directly related to the physical or mental condition of the individual, since the availability of informal carers affects the need for domiciliary services and residential care, as discussed later. The marital status of older people is the principal determinant of their living arrangements, and therefore of the availability of other household members to provide informal care should this be needed. Because of men's higher mortality (Table 8.1) and the cultural norm of men marrying women younger than themselves, women can expect to be widowed for 8–10 years. Half of women over age 65 are widowed, mostly living alone, while nearly three-quarters of older men are married (Arber & Ginn 1991). A third factor is that health-care costs may be inflated by socially constructed illnesses (Robertson 1991), due to the 'biomedicalisation of ageing', as we discuss later.

Concern in the media and by policy makers with 'demographic facts' about the increasing size of the elderly population reflects contemporary ageism and reinforces stereotypes of older people as a burden and a separate group from the rest of society (Bytheway 1995). Since the majority of older people, especially the very old, are women, this concern is sexist as well as ageist.

Ageism and the NHS

As well as the ageism inherent in contemporary society, it is important to consider whether health providers are explicitly or implicitly ageist in their priorities, and if so, how this might affect older people. Henwood states 'not only is there widespread discrimination against older people in the provision of health care, but they are also the victims of restricted assumptions about the quality of health care which can be expected in old age' (1990: 43).

How care is rationed and to what extent chronological age is or should be a criterion for provision of medical procedures are matters of increasing urgency, yet they are seldom articulated. Approaches based on quality adjusted life years (QALYs), are increasingly advocated, but these are inherently age-discriminatory in two ways (Henwood 1990). First, counting extra years as part of the benefit of medical procedures risks shifting resources away from older to younger age groups. Second, those judged to have a low quality of life, predominantly older people, will be disadvantaged.

The provision of health care in the 1990s has been dominated by a concern to achieve the objectives specified in *The Health of the Nation* (Department of Health 1992). However, this provides little comfort for older people, because the emphasis is on reducing 'premature death'.

The main targets specify upper age limits, for example, to reduce rates of coronary heart disease (CHD) and stroke among those under 65 and 65–74, and to reduce lung cancer under the age of 75. Since CHD and stroke are the major causes of death among women and men over 75, exclusion from such targets is discriminatory. Only one target specifically mentions older people, and this is to reduce the death rate from accidents among people over 65. This target may be considered of particular benefit to the NHS, since setting broken bones and the rehabilitation costs following accidents form a major part of NHS expenditure.

Screening programmes may also have age criteria which are discriminatory (Henwood 1990). Women aged 65 and over are denied routine screening for cervical cancer, yet 40% of deaths from cancer of the cervix occur in women over 65. Similarly, breast screening programmes have a maximum age of 64, although pilot studies are currently being carried out on women over 65 in various parts of Britain. However, other programmes target older people for screening: GPs are now required to offer an annual check up for all patients aged 75 and over. Therefore some age-based criteria for screening tend to suggest that diagnosing and treating older people's cancers is a low priority, while others reinforce the conflation of old age with incapacity and generalised ill health.

A critical area in which older people have been largely excluded is epidemiological studies and trials of clinical interventions, so that the effects of therapies on older people are unknown (MRC 1994). This could lead to clinicians making inappropriate decisions, adversely affecting older people's health. The MRC recommend that in future research studies should have no upper age limit: 'Older people have the potential to benefit directly from therapeutic and preventive health care strategies, and often stand to benefit proportionately more than their juniors from technological advances' and that 'Age should not, therefore, be the sole criterion for the exclusion of older people from medical and surgical interventions generally made more available to younger people. Rather, emphasis should be on physiological status and not chronological age to determine health care' (p. 62).

The process of normal ageing has been increasingly brought within the medical paradigm, in which it is constructed as pathological, a medical problem which can be treated and cured (Robertson 1991). 'The equation of old age with illness has encouraged society to think about ageing as pathological or abnormal.' (Estes & Binney 1991: 118). This 'biomedicalisation of ageing' focuses attention on the diseases of older people, their aetiology, treatment and management from the perspective of doctors. It tends to neglect the ways in which social, environmental and behavioural factors influence the process and experience of ageing.

In particular, there is a danger of overzealous curative treatment, irrespective of the older patient's wishes, especially in the professional project to defy death.

The medicalisation of ageing and death may increase the dependency of older people on medical experts, subjecting them to social control; it may also increase health care expenditure. The emphasis on clinical problems and medically defined solutions to the 'problems of ageing' has neglected the concerns of older people. Health providers need to shift from a focus in which older people are seen primarily as medical problems to one which sees them as subjects rather than objects, allowing them to define their own health needs, priorities and concerns.

Gender inequalities in health among older people

Most older women and men are healthy, live independently and provide for their own self-care. Good health, especially the capacity to carry out personal self-care, such as bathing, eating, negotiating stairs and walking outside the home, is essential to independence. Chronic illness and disability tend to restrict independence, as well as generating extra costs for a special diet, additional heating, laundry, or nursing care and necessitating practical support and personal care from informal carers or the state.

Health is a major concern of older people, and their key concern is that they should not become dependent on others due to deteriorating health. Older women are more likely than older men to suffer from conditions which are non-fatal but result in chronic and disabling illnesses which hinder their activities of daily living. In 1985, 7% of men and 14% of women over 65 suffered from disabilities serious enough to require help on a daily basis to remain living in the community (Arber & Ginn, 1991).

The 1994 General Household Survey confirmed the gender difference in functional abilities (Bennett *et al.* 1996). Under one-fifth of men over 85 were unable to go out and walk down the road, compared with nearly half of women. Less than 10% of men over 85 were unable to go up and downstairs, compared with 29% of women. The levels of mobility restrictions were low for men and women aged 65–74, with the likelihood of a mobility restriction increasing markedly above age 85. In terms of personal self-care, 10% of women over 65 and 6% of men were unable to bath, shower or wash all over without assistance but this restriction applied to nearly one-quarter of women over 85. Inability to do household shopping largely reflects inability to walk far outside, which was the case for one-fifth of women and one-tenth of men over 65, rising to over half of women over 85 and one-quarter of men over 85. Therefore, although most older people can live independently, older women are more likely to suffer from disabling conditions which mean they require help from others in the community or from state services.

Material resources in later life

When considering older people, it is essential to analyse material resources such as income, assets, car ownership, housing and the quality of the home environment, and how they interrelate with the bodily resources of physical health and functional abilities, as well as access to personal, social and health care (Arber & Ginn 1991). These interlinked sets of resources influence an older person's level of independence, sense of autonomy, capacity for sociability and involvement in leisure pursuits. The absence of any one of these resources acts as a constraint on well-being, sapping morale and increasing their likelihood of dependency.

An adequate income is vital to the health of older people. Not only is it necessary to provide the basic health needs of heating, an adequate diet and decent housing, but it is also increasingly important because of the growing need to pay for social and health care. An adequate income maximises the likelihood of an older person maintaining independence within a given level of disability, by allowing the purchase of home aids and adaptations, moving to more suitable accommodation, or paying for private transport when required. Cutbacks in public transport reduce opportunities for social and leisure activities and may increase social isolation. The effects on older women have been particularly severe, because they are less likely to drive or to have sufficient financial resources to run a car.

Government policies over the last 15 years have increased income inequality among older people by reducing the value of state National Insurance pensions. In 1996, the state pension was under £5000 p.a. for a married couple and £3076 p.a. for an unmarried older person – below the means-tested Income Support level. The worst effects have been felt by older women, because of their greater reliance on state pensions. In 1991, the median personal income of older men was £106 per week, the top 25% (upper quartile) receiving over £180 per week, whereas older women's personal income fell far below men's, with a median of only £61 and an upper quartile of £91 per week (Arber & Ginn 1994). This gender inequality of income stems mainly from women's lower receipt of occupational and personal pensions, due to the constraints placed on their employment pattern, occupational level and lifetime earnings by unpaid domestic and caring work (Ginn & Arber 1993, 1996). Thus two-thirds of older men, but only a quarter of older women, have an occupational or personal pension and the amounts of these pensions are considerably lower for women (Arber & Ginn 1994). Older people are much poorer in Britain than in most other western European countries (Walker & Maltby, 1997).

Class and income inequalities in health

There has been less research on class inequalities in health among older people than at other stages of the life course. This reflects both the tendency to see older people as a homogeneous group and the difficulties of measuring class for older people (Arber & Ginn 1993). Class is sometimes considered problematic to measure for older people, who have generally left the labour market many years earlier. For older women, the conventional approach of classifying them by their husband's occupational class is impossible, because half of older women are widowed. Despite these problems, our work has shown that class based on the older person's last main occupation reveals clear class gradients in health (Arber & Ginn 1993, Arber 1996).

To illustrate the persistence of structural inequalities in health in later life, Table 8.2 shows the results of logistic regression analyses of class and income differences in self-assessed health based on the General Household Survey for 1991–93. Self-assessed health is measured by the question; 'Over the last 12 months, would you say your health has on the whole been good, fairly good or not good?' The separate models for men and women over 65 in each case control for marital status and 5-year age groups.

Odds ratios of 'less than good health' by occupational class are shown in the first and fourth columns of Table 8.2. For both older men and women there is a linear class gradient; men previously in semi- or unskilled occupations had over twice the odds ratio of reporting 'less than good' health compared with men who had previously been in higher non-manual occupations (the reference category). Class differences for women show a manual/non-manual divide, with older women who previously worked in a manual occupation having a 50% higher odds ratio than women who previously worked in a non-manual job.

Tenure is a strong predictor of health, older women and men living in public housing have almost twice the odds ratio of reporting poor health compared with those who own their homes. When housing tenure is

Table 8.2   Odds ratios of 'less than good' health for men and women aged 65 and over.

	Men			Women		
	+ Social class	+ Housing tenure	+ Income	+ Social class	+ Housing tenure	+ Income
Social Class	+++	+++	+	+++	++	+
Higher non-manual	1.00	1.00	1.00	1.00	1.00	1.00
Junior non-manual	1.48**	1.36*	1.23	0.99	0.96	0.94
Skilled manual	1.97**	1.67**	1.35**	1.53**	1.36*	1.26
Semi-skilled	2.36**	1.85**	1.51**	1.54**	1.29*	1.20
Unskilled	2.16**	1.63*	1.33	1.69**	1.32*	1.21
Never worked				1.20	1.15	1.13
Housing tenure		+++	+++		+++	+++
Owner occupier		1.00	1.00		1.00	1.00
Public rental		1.89**	1.64**		1.97**	1.77**
Other rental		1.16	1.07		1.28	1.18
Income			+++			++
Upper 20%			1.00			1.00
60% < 80%			1.61**			1.16
40% < 60%			1.66**			1.32*
20% < 40%			2.07**			1.34*
Lowest 20%			1.91**			1.59**
Change in LLR	69.7	41.1	30.6	42.9	72.4	15.1
Change in df	4	2	4	5	2	4
Significance of change	p<.001	p<.001	p<.001	p<.001	p<.001	p<.01
N =	2593			3565		

Source: General Household Survey, 1991/92 and 1992/93 (authors' analysis).

Base model includes age in five year age groups and marital status
LLR - LogLikelihood ratio; df - degrees of freedom.
+++ Significance of variable in the model, +++ p<0.001, ++ p<0.01, + p<0.05.
** Significance of difference from reference category, ** p<0.01, * p<0.05.

included in the models (second and fifth columns), the strength of the class gradient is somewhat diminished but remains statistically significant.

Level of income is clearly related to the health of older people, even after social class and housing tenure are included in the model (columns 3 and 6). The effect of income is especially pronounced for older men; men in the lowest 40% of the income distribution have nearly twice the odds ratio of poor health compared with men receiving the top 20% of income. The effects of income on older women's self-perceived health are not as strong as for men. Although inclusion of income and housing tenure in the models reduces social class inequalities in health, class remains statistically significant for older men. Our analysis demonstrates the continuing importance of the nature of previous employment for the current health of older people. Occupational class during working life influences both an older person's level of income and their housing tenure, but each of these three factors has an independent effect on their health, especially for men.

The availability of family carers

Changes in community care policies in the early 1990s made it more difficult for older people to obtain Local Authority-funded residential care and home care (Walker 1993). Although such policies are put forward as gender-neutral, the adverse effects have been greater for older women. First, older men have more financial resources to pay for care, as discussed earlier. Second, older women are more likely than men to have a functional disability. Third, men are more likely to have a wife who can provide care should they need it, whereas older women tend to live alone (Arber & Ginn 1991, 1995). Older disabled women are twice as likely as men with a comparable level of disability to live alone and therefore are more reliant than men on family members living elsewhere, other informal carers in the community, and state provided domiciliary services. Nearly two-thirds of severely disabled older men can rely on support/care provided by their wife. Severely disabled older women are twice as likely as equivalent men to live in the home of an adult child.

When older disabled people share their household with others, household members perform virtually all of the necessary personal and domestic care tasks for them, and state services are provided at a very low level. However, care from family members, from different providers in the community, and from the state may not be equally acceptable from the older person's point of view, having different implications for their self-esteem and degree of autonomy.

The greatest threat to an older person's autonomy and independence is generally considered to be entry into a nursing or residential home. Despite the expansion of private residential homes during the 1980s, the 1991 population census showed that only 3% of men and 6.4% of women over 65 lived in communal establishments (OPCS 1993), an increase from 2.5% of men and 4.6% of women in 1981 (Arber & Ginn 1991). The gender differential in communal residence is greater above age 80, and is particularly pronounced over age 85, when 26% of women and 15% of men are residents.

An older person's marital status has a very significant effect on their likelihood of living in a residential setting (Fig. 8.1). The greater proportion of older women than men living in residential settings primarily reflects their higher likelihood of being widowed, and without a

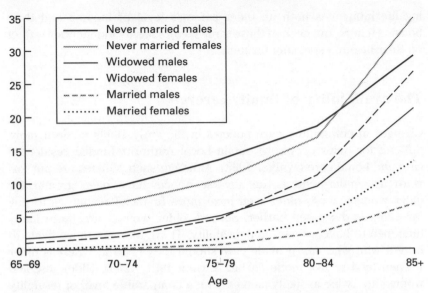

Source: OPCS (1994) *Census 1991, Communal Establishments, Great Britain,* London: HMSO, Table 2.

Fig. 8.1 Percentage of older men and women resident in communal establishments in 1991, by marital status and age groups.

partner to care for them should they become disabled. Residential care is most likely for never married men and least likely for married men and women, in each age group. For example, in the 65–69 age group, only 0.2% of the married live in a communal establishment compared with 8% of single men and 6% of single women: thus, the single are over 30 times more likely than the married to live in a residential setting. There is a tenfold advantage of the married compared with the never married in their late seventies, and even among those over 85, four times more single (29%) than married men (7%) live in residential care, and three times more single (35%) than married women (13%) live in a residential setting. The widowed are in an intermediate position in each age group.

Marital status can be interpreted as a proxy for the availability of family carers, with the marital differential in residential living demonstrating the very substantial role played by informal carers in supporting older people in the community. Never married people are least likely to have family carers, the widowed and divorced generally have children as potential carers, while for married older people their partner is likely to be their carer, unless they are too frail or disabled to perform this role.

Conclusions: ageing and the policy context

Current attitudes discriminate against older people, neglect their socially useful work and see them as an unproductive burden rather than as contributors to society. Over a third of informal care for older people is provided by people over age 65, mainly older spouses caring for their disabled partner, as well as those caring for neighbours and friends (Arber & Ginn 1991). Older people are the backbone of voluntary support in the health service and innumerable other organisations; without their unpaid work, such organisations would have to recruit additional paid staff or provide poorer quality services. A major source of childcare for the increasing proportion of working women is their own mother or mother-in-law. The characterisation of older people as an unproductive burden is not only inaccurate, but has been used to justify cuts in state pensions and services for older people.

The use of exclusionary terms like 'the elderly' draws an implicit contrast between 'us', the non-elderly – the normal, and 'them', the elderly – the 'other'. Such terms reinforce perceptions of older people as a distinctive group, which Bytheway (1995) argues characterise older people as a 'burden en bloc'. To portray older people in this negative light is not only ageist but sexist, since women are numerically dominant in later life. Thus, ageist concerns about the burdens of the very old primarily pathologise older women, who form the majority of the very frail and especially those in need of care by the state or informal carers.

Discussions which scapegoat older people, whether framed as apocalyptic demography or in terms of intergenerational equity, deflect attention from other sources of strain on the public purse: unemployment, tax relief for private welfare insurance and the medicalisation of dying. They also ignore social changes which could reduce the cost of care for older people in future. In considering the reasons for the chorus of opposition to welfare spending on older people, it is worth remembering that powerful interest groups profit from private pensions and health care and that these businesses thrive on the perceived run-down of publicly provided welfare such as the NHS in Britain.

The progressively earlier age of exit from paid employment and improving health of the population has meant that women and men spend many more active years not in paid work, both before and after the state pension age, than in the past. The British state pension, which was introduced after the Second World War, has made it possible for older people to live independently of both paid work and of financial support from relatives. However, current trends in social and economic policy are threatening to reverse these gains, particularly for older women.

The greater the movement towards individual provision for retirement through occupational and personal pensions, the greater will be the income inequality between older women and men and between those with an intermittent, or low paid employment history and those with an advantaged position in the labour market. Current government policies relating to pensions are leading to growing inequality among older people according to their previous occupation and the continuity of their employment career. Thus the opportunities to enjoy a Third Age of self-development and autonomous action are likely to become increasingly gendered, as well as class-divided, with financial dependency acting as an obstacle to citizenship rights (Arber & Ginn 1995). We showed how low income is associated with poor health. Thus, the health consequences of the growing income inequality among older people should not be ignored.

Although older women have a longer expectation of life than men, they also have a longer period in which they can expect to be disabled or live in a residential setting. The gender differential in disability means that older women are more likely to require both informal care and state health and welfare services. Nearly half of disabled older women live alone, which while promoting independence means they are reliant on state domiciliary services, mainly home care services and community nurses. They are also heavily dependent on the unpaid work of relatives and other informal carers, and are more likely to enter residential care. Older women's disadvantage is compounded by their lower average income; a poor deal for the majority of women who have spent a lifetime of unpaid work looking after children, husband and others, often in addition to waged work.

An increasingly salient health issue for older people is whether they will have any control over the timing and manner of their own death, should they suffer a painful or debilitating terminal illness. With longer life and higher expectations of personal choice and autonomy than in the past, public campaigns to legalise voluntary euthanasia and debate about the social, ethical, legal and medical questions around euthanasia are growing (Glick 1996). Given the prevalence of ageist portrayals of older people as a burden, a concern that older people should not feel pressured into ending their life when ill or disabled is understandable. Nevertheless, it would be a perverse outcome from their point of view if this concern were to prevent the search for suitably safeguarded ways to enable those who wish it to 'die with dignity'.

In an NHS increasingly concerned about rationing health resources, the danger is that rationing care according to chronological age will become more overt. This would have a greater detrimental effect on women, who form the majority of the very old. Policies of community care, which have restricted access to state-funded domicilary and residential care, have been particularly disadvantageous for older women because of their longevity and greater chance of being widowed.

Sociologists need to give older women and men a voice, and to provide them with an opportunity to define the health issues of relevance to them. We need to move their personal concerns and priorities to centre-stage, seeing older people as the subjects rather than the objects of health research. Finally, we need to be sensitive to the relationship between structural inequalities and health among older people, in particular how material and social resources in later life are shaped by gender and class, and how these have been fashioned by earlier phases of their personal biography.

Acknowledgements

We are to grateful to the Office of National Statistics for permission to use data from the General Household Survey, and to the Data Archive and Manchester Computing Centre for access to the data. We are grateful to Tom Daly for the analysis of residential care.

References

Arber, S. (1996) Integrating non-employment into research on health inequalities. *International Journal of Health Services*, **26**, 445–81.

Arber, S. & Ginn, J. (1991) *Gender and Later Life: A Sociological Analysis of Resources and Constraints*. Sage, London.

Arber, S. & Ginn, J. (1993) Gender and inequalities in health in later life. *Social Science and Medicine*, **36**, 33–46.

Arber, S. & Ginn, J. (1994) Women and ageing. *Reviews in Clinical Gerontology*, **4**, 93–102.

Arber, S. & Ginn, J. (1995) *Connecting Gender and Ageing: A Sociological Approach*. Open University Press, Buckingham.

Bennett, N., Jarvis, L. & Rowlands, O. (1996) *Living in Britain: Results of the 1994 General Household Survey, OPCS*. HMSO, London.

Bytheway, B. (1995) *Ageism*, Open University Press, Buckingham.

Central Statistical Office (1996) *Social Trends 1996*. HMSO, London.

Department of Health (1992) *The Health of the Nation: A Strategy for Health in England*, Cmd 1986. HMSO, London.

Estes, C. & Binney, E. (1991) The biomedicalization of aging: dangers and dilemmas. In: *Critical Perspectives on Gerontology: The Political and Moral Economy of Growing Old* (eds M. Minkler & C. Estes), pp. 117–34. Baywood, New York.

Featherstone, M. & Hepworth, M. (1989) Ageing and old age: reflections on the postmodern lifecourse. In: *Becoming and Being Old: Sociological Approaches to Later Life* (eds B. Bytheway, T. Keil, P. Allatt & A. Bryman), pp. 143–57. Sage, London.

Featherstone, M. & Hepworth, M. (1991) The mask of ageing and the postmodern life course. In: *The Body: Social Process and Cultural Theory* (eds M. Featherstone, M. Hepworth & B.S. Turner), pp. 371–89. Sage, London.

Fries, J. (1989) Reduction of the national morbidity. In: *Aging and Health* (ed. S. Lewis), pp. 3–22. Lewis, Michigan.

Ginn, J. & Arber, S. (1993) Pension penalties: the gendered division of occupational welfare. *Work, Employment and Society*, **7**, 47–70.

Ginn, J. & Arber, S. (1996) Patterns of employment, gender and pensions: the effect of work history on older women's non-state pensions. *Work, Employment and Society*, **10**, 469–90.

Glick, H. (1996) Death, technology and politics. In: *Aging for the Twenty-first Century* (eds J. Quadagno & D. Street), pp. 549–67. St Martin's Press, New York.

Green, H. (1988) *Informal Carers*, OPCS Series GHS, No. 15, Supplement A, OPCS. HMSO, London.

Henwood, M. (1990) No sense of urgency: Age discrimination in health care. In: *Age: The Unrecognised Discrimination* (ed. E. McEwen), pp. 43–57. Age Concern, London.

Laslett, P. (1989) *A Fresh Map of Life: The Emergence of the Third Age*. Weidenfeld and Nicolson, London.

Lewis, J. & Meredith, B. (1988) *Daughters Who Care*. Routledge, London.

Manton, K.G., Stallard, E. & Corder, L. (1995) Changes in morbidity and chronic disability in the U.S. elderly population: evidence from the 1982, 1984 and 1989 National Long Term Care Survey. *Journal of Gerontology*, **50B**, S104–S204.

Medical Research Council (1994) *The Health of the UK's Elderly People*. MRC, London.

Meredeen, S. (1995) The seven stages of Shirley Meredeen. In: *Disgracefully Yours: Inspirational Writings for Growing Older – and Living Life to the Full!* (eds The Hen Co-op), pp. 54–5. Judy Piatkins (Publishers) Ltd, London.

Minkler, M. (1991) 'Generational equity' and the new victim blaming. In: *Critical Perspectives on Gerontology: The Political and Moral Economy of Growing Old* (eds M. Minkler & C. Estes), pp. 67–80. Baywood, New York.

OPCS (1993) *Communal Establishments, 1991 Census*. HMSO, London.

Robertson, A. (1991) The politics of Alzheimer's disease: A case study on apocalyptic demography. In: *Critical Perspectives on Gerontology: The Political and Moral Economy of Growing Old* (eds M. Minkler & C. Estes), pp. 135–54. Baywood, New York.

Verbrugge, L. (1989) The dynamics of population aging and health. In: *Aging and Health* (ed. S. Lewis), pp. 23–40. Lewis, Michigan.

Walker, A. (1993) Community care policy: From consensus to conflict. In: *Community Care: A Reader* (eds J. Bornat, C. Pereira, D. Pilgrim & F. Williams), pp. 204–226. Macmillan, London.

Walker, A. & Maltby, T. (1997) *Ageing Europe*. Open University Press, Buckingham.

Part III
The Provision of Health Care

Chapter 9
The Politics of Health Care Reform in Britain: A Moving Consensus?

Rob Baggott

Introduction

The partisan nature of debates about health care reform creates difficulties for those seeking to analyse policy making in this area. In particular, the rhetoric adopted by political parties often distorts the true extent of agreement and disagreement between them, understating the degree to which they are prepared to compromise on their ideals in practice. In order to achieve a better understanding of the dynamics of health policy one has to move beyond rhetoric to focus on actual policy changes and consider the processes which promote and inhibit policy development.

The concept of political consensus provides a useful framework for such an analysis, as it relates not only to policy debates but to political processes and ultimately to changes and continuities in policy itself. Political consensus is usually characterised simply as agreement on policy or 'policy coincidence' between political parties and among interest groups involved in a particular policy arena. Yet a high degree of policy coincidence is only one of several aspects of political consensus (Smith 1979). Others include an open and consultative style of policy making, which facilitates the incorporation of organised interests (Kavanagh 1985), and a political process which promotes policy continuity and incrementalism. These features, though not preventing policy innovation, discriminate in favour of initiatives which have at least the potential to become more widely accepted. In other words even radical policies can become part of a moving consensus, as described by Rose and Davies (1995):

'In addition to adopting programs that have bipartisan support, each administration is likely to promote some choices to which it gives a high priority but which do not have bipartisan endorsement at the moment of their introduction . The opposition may vote against these programs, but once in office it will accept what it has inherited. Instead of being repealed, new programs will be incorporated into a moving consensus.'   (p. 125)

In this chapter we examine these various aspects of political consensus in the context of health care reform.

Policy coincidence

In the 1950s and 1960s health issues had a relatively low political profile. The Conservative minister Macleod, writing in 1958, claimed that with the exception of the issue of charges, health was 'out of party politics' (quoted in Klein 1995: 29). An initial reaction is that these comments could not be applied to recent decades, where the public division between the major parties has been all too evident. A more critical approach requires examination of the extent of policy coincidence in the pre-Thatcher era and to ask whether the degree of policy differences in the 1980s and 1990s has been exaggerated.

Post-war consensus?

There is evidence that the Conservative governments of the 1950s and 1960s were willing to consider policy options that explicitly challenged the post-war consensus on health. For example, the establishment of the Guillebaud Committee in 1952, to inquire into the cost of the NHS, represented an attempt not only to squeeze funding but to restrict the scope of the service. In the event the Committee asserted its independence, identified a shortfall in funding, and strengthened rather than undermined the case for a comprehensive national health service (Cmd. 9663 1956, Webster 1988). Later in the decade, the Conservatives actively considered, though in a secretive and fairly cautious way, a range of highly controversial measures which if implemented would have undermined the post-war consensus on the NHS. These included scrapping free NHS dental services, hotel charges for patients and charging for visits to the GP (Webster 1994, 1996). Alternative ways of funding the NHS, including a compulsory national insurance scheme, were also explored.

During the 1950s and 1960s Conservative governments did increase national insurance contributions and charges for prescriptions and other items. Moreover, according to Webster (1994), the NHS was starved of resources in this period in such a way as to prevent the emergence of the range and quality of care intended by its creators. However, the more radical ideas were not carried forward, largely for electoral reasons. The fear of hostile public reaction to policies perceived as undermining the NHS or restricting its scope in effect maintained the broad consensus described by Macleod. Partisan battles over the NHS did take place in the House of Commons, but were mainly rhetorical set pieces reflecting adversarial Parliamentary traditions and the rigidities of the 'two-party' system, which was at its height in this period.

The broad public consensus between the major parties kept ideological tendencies in check throughout the latter part of the 1960s and into the 1970s. This was a period in which the political pendulum swung back to Labour. The degree of consensus was demonstrated by the reorganisation of the NHS, a process which both major parties saw as a necessary step (Klein 1995: 83). The reorganisation evolved over a six-year period beginning with Labour's policy proposals in 1968 and 1970. Further consultations were undertaken by the incoming Conservative administration of 1970–74, which modified the plans within the broad principles of reorganisation set out by its predecessor, and steered through the necessary legislation. The reorganisation was finally implemented by a Labour Government in 1974.

However, this measure was not without controversy. Despite the agreement between the two main parties on the broad principles of reorganisation, they vociferously attacked each others' proposals. Yet although the passage of the NHS reorganisation bill in the Commons was dominated by a partisan-ideological approach, health policy was increasingly becoming a technical rather than a partisan matter (Ingle & Tether 1981). So the posturing of the parties had little impact on policy, which was largely shaped by other factors such as the views of interest groups and expert advisors, as well as practical and technical constraints.

Throughout the 1970s, there were signs that the consensus surrounding health policy was beginning to unravel. In particular the 1974–79 Labour government's policy on pay beds in the NHS was seen as a challenge to the post-war settlement. Klein (1995: 106), for example, maintains that the battle over private beds was different because it threatened the consensus which had prevailed since the creation of the NHS. Doctors protested that their rights to private practice – an important concession made by the state back in 1946 to win the profession's support – were being curtailed. But even on this controversial issue a compromise was eventually reached. The Prime Minister, Harold Wilson, appointed an intermediary, Lord Goodman, to help negotiate a solution to the crisis. This led to the creation of the Health Services Board which sought to reduce rather than abolish pay beds. But even this fairly modest arrangement failed to survive a change of government. The Conservatives, who had supported the doctors in the pay beds dispute, abolished the Health Services Board in 1980.

The 1970s brought economic crises, which undermined the ability of the state to fund the NHS in line with rising expectations. This brought the Labour government into conflict with the NHS workforce and provided plenty of ammunition for the Conservative opposition. For example, in a debate on the NHS in 1975 the shadow spokesman for social services, Norman Fowler, highlighted the underfunding of the NHS in terms that would not have disgraced his Labour successor.

'Lack of resources means that new hospitals cannot be built, that much-needed extensions cannot go ahead and that new equipment cannot be bought.... that medical staff are working in conditions that no-one can consider ideal and that are often blatantly inadequate ... that nurses who finish their training are unable to find posts in the hospitals in which they have trained, not because they are not needed, but because there is no money to employ them.'   (Fowler 1975)

At the same time, the Conservative opposition acknowledged that there were no simple solutions to the funding problems of the NHS. It placed its faith in reorganisation and management reform, and was reluctant to commit extra resources to the service. So in this respect at least, rather than a declining consensus about NHS funding, there was in fact a growing understanding among the leaders of all parties that a tougher line on public expenditure on health care would be necessary.

Thatcherism

Although significant policy disagreements preceded the election of the Thatcher government in 1979, there had been no serious challenge to the dominant collectivist philosophy underpinning the NHS, with its emphasis upon public provision, tax-funded services, and its principles of universality and equality of access. Once in power, however, the Conservative government began to explore the possibility of health reforms that reflected new right (or neo-liberal) philosophy. This philosophy was based on very different principles, including: a minimal state, hostility to bureaucracy and organised labour (including the professions), endorsement of market mechanisms, private enterprise and private sector management methods, empowerment of individual consumers, the promotion of self-reliance and voluntarism (Green 1987). According to the new right perspective in its pure form, health care could be regarded much as any other good or service, and should be subject to allocation by consumer choice as expressed through the market.

From the early 1980s onwards these ideals began to be reflected in policies, such as the Griffiths management reforms, the NHS internal market, the community care reforms, market testing, the Private Finance Initiative and the encouragement of private health care. The government's endorsement of these principles also foreclosed many options regarded as vital by some, but which went against the grain of the neo-liberal philosophy, as exemplified by the government's rejection throughout the 1980s and 1990s of a strategy to combat health inequalities and its reluctance to tackle the commercial and industrial sources of ill health.

Although 'new right' principles exerted an important influence on health policy in the 1980s and into the following decade, it would be wrong to see them as totally dominant. Other factors also shaped health policy in this period. The collectivist ideology in health care proved very durable and this is perhaps why, as Wistow (1992) observed, the basic principles of the NHS were able to survive the Thatcher governments. Even Margaret Thatcher herself denied that she sought to undermine these principles:

'Although I wanted to see a flourishing private sector of health alongside the National Health Service, I always regarded the NHS and its basic principles as a fixed point in our policies.'

(Thatcher 1993: 606)

Though some may doubt these words, it is nevertheless the case that the Thatcher governments were often on the defensive in discussions about the future of the NHS and made great efforts to reassure the public that its health policies would not harm the service. This occurred most famously in 1982, with Thatcher's declaration – following the leak of an internal review outlining the scope for privatisation in the NHS – that 'the National Health Service is safe with us' (Thatcher 1982). Later, prior to the introduction of the internal market in the NHS in 1991, the government sought to reassure the public by avoiding wherever possible commercial language when referring to the new policy. Furthermore, ministers subsequently used their powers to intervene in the internal market in a number of ways, for example, restricting the commercial freedom of the self-governing trusts, attempting to strengthen frameworks of planning and accountability, and introducing guidance governing admissions to hospital in response to concerns about the development of a 'two-tier' system.

During the 1980s attitude surveys revealed growing public dissatisfaction with the NHS. This was interpreted by some as a signal that the public were losing faith in the service. In 1983, 26% of the population claimed to be quite or very dissatisfied with the NHS. This rose to 47% in 1990, declining subsequently to 38% in 1993 (Bosanquet 1994). However, overall public support for the NHS did not decline. Instead, there was considerable hostility to reforms which appeared to undermine its fundamental principles. Attitude surveys indicated that the NHS remained one of the most popular public services and that in spite of the growth of private health insurance, health care was still seen by the public as primarily the state's responsibility. Moreover, there was a strong opposition to the idea of a 'two-tier' health care system, where the NHS caters mainly for the uninsured (Bosanquet 1994).

The public consensus underpinning the NHS insulated it to some extent from the application of new right principles. So that although Conservative health care reforms reflected these principles, in practice there was a compromise with pre-existing collectivist values. Furthermore, some of the health policies pursued by the Thatcher and Major governments were not exclusively based on new right principles. Policies directed at empowering individuals, encouraging voluntarism and self-help, and making professions more accountable to those whom they serve, attracted support from across the political spectrum. Indeed, many of the criticisms of contemporary health care employed by the new right, in particular those relating to the power of producers relative to consumers, had been previously raised by others (e.g. Illich 1975, Kennedy 1981). Moreover, many policies introduced in the 1980s and 1990s had origins in the period before the ascendancy of the new right. For example, the introduction of general management into the NHS was advocated by reformers back in the 1960s.

The impact of the new right upon health policy was mitigated further by tensions between its key principles. Important conflicts of principle arose between managerialism and the notion of the 'minimal state'. Managerialism is essentially an authoritarian approach, which emphasises centralisation, command and control, whereas the minimal state concept implies a smaller role for central government, decentralisation of power and considerable autonomy for front-line workers. This tension was particularly noticeable in relation to policies which sought to off-load functions into the private sector and those which attempted to retain control. Hence the guidance issued by government in the early 1980s allowing consultants to do more private work, inhibited efforts later in the decade to exert more managerial control over them. Conflicts in practice also emerged, even between principles which appeared consistent. Take, for example, the principles of marketisation and anti-bureaucracy. In practice the creation of markets in health care generated an increase in the NHS bureaucracy, both in terms of staffing (the number of NHS managers increased fourfold between 1989–94) and workload (i.e. an increase in form-filling and paperwork associated with performance measures and the internal market in particular) with implications for the overall efficiency of the service.

Pragmatism

These conflicts weakened the overall impact of the new right perspective, creating a vacuum which was filled by a more pragmatic response to the problems of health care. For example, after initially denying that recent policies had generated a growth in NHS bureaucracy, the Major government later embarked on a drive to cut management costs and paperwork. In general, more pragmatic responses emerged as health policies began to generate political and practical problems. As will become clear later, these problems were particularly acute at the policy implementation stage.

During the 1980s and 1990s, in spite of the rhetoric, Conservative governments often demonstrated a great deal of pragmatism, and on occasion showed a willingness to adopt proposals from other sources. On entering office in 1979, the Thatcher government accepted some of the recommendations made by the Royal Commission on the NHS, created by previous Labour government. Moreover, the Major and Thatcher governments were often defensive and reactive in the field of health policy, the agenda being influenced by opposition parties, pressure groups and the media.

The Conservatives even borrowed policy ideas directly from other political parties. For example, the Labour and Liberal Parties supported the idea of a Patient's Charter long before the Conservatives introduced their own version in 1992. Similarly, the idea of a national health strategy was promoted by the opposition parties well in advance of the Conservatives' Health of the Nation proposals launched in 1991. True, the Conservative's policies differed considerably in detail from those advanced by the opposition parties – for example the Health of the Nation strategy ignored health inequalities, socio-economic factors and commercial and industrial causes of ill health. Nevertheless, the extent to which the Conservatives were prepared to steal their opponents' clothes revealed a much more flexible policy process. This was further exemplified by the acceptance of key parts of the Conservative government's programme of reform by the opposition parties.

The discussion so far reveals that trends in health policy are more complex than they first appear. In the 1950s and 1960s there was a high

degree of consensus – in terms of agreement in public on policy issues –
although policies with the potential to undermine this were actively, if
secretly, under consideration. In the 1970s, there was evidence of a
weakening consensus, which was accentuated in the 1980s as the
Thatcher government adopted alternative ideological reference points.
However, in practice the strong underlying public consensus inhibited
radical policy change, limiting the extent to which the Conservative
government could actually manoeuvre. The situation was complicated
further by tensions and conflicts between the new right principles,
examined above, which in some situations led to a policy vacuum.
Meanwhile, other actors, such as the opposition parties, the media and
pressure groups, shaped policy by promoting their ideas and concerns
on the political agenda and, as will become clear in the next section, by
exposing flaws in policy at the implementation stage.

Policy style

Although the Conservative governments of the 1980s and 1990s depar-
ted from new right principles when implementing health policies, the
impression remains that they nevertheless undermined consensus by
an authoritarian approach to health policy making. For most of the
post-war period, as in most other areas of domestic policy making,
consultation before legislation became an established principle of government. The use of independent committees of inquiry, which gath-
ered evidence before putting forward their recommendations in a
published report, was one manifestation of this. Hence the Guillebaud
committee was able to assert its independence and so frustrate the
intentions of its creators. However, confrontation was not entirely
absent, as the dispute between the government and general practitioners (GPs) over pay and conditions in 1965 clearly illustrated. The
GPs threatened to resign from the NHS if their demands were not met
– though eventually the issue was settled through negotiation. Moving
into the 1970s such confrontations became routine, part of a national
trend of industrial conflict. Nevertheless all the main disputes in this
period were eventually settled by compromise and negotiation, including the controversial pay beds issue.

If anything, the evidence points to a strengthening of consultative
processes in the 1970s. This is illustrated by the Labour government's
appointment of a Royal Commission in 1976 to examine the problems
facing the NHS. The Royal Commission (Cmd 7615 1979) received evidence from a wide range of sources, spent three years discussing the
problems of the service and possible solutions. It made 117 recom-

mendations, some of which were implemented by the incoming Conservative administration, notably the removal of an operational tier of NHS administration, the creation of a limited list of NHS medicines, an extension of screening programmes, and medical audit.

Thatcher's style of government

This broadly consensual approach to health policy making contrasted with the Thatcher government's policy style during the 1980s, which was for the most part centralised, closed and secretive. For example, the NHS internal market, announced in 1989, was initiated by a small group of ministers and special advisors headed by the Prime Minister. The policy process was closed in that, as Butler (1992: 5) observes, it 'had no public terms of reference and no formal consultations were held'. Specially selected groups of doctors and managers were consulted at two private meetings, but not in a representative capacity. Organised interests – the trade unions and professional organisations – were permitted to submit their proposals for reform through the Department of Health, but not allowed to put their case directly to the review.

However, not all health policy initiatives introduced by the Conservatives during the 1980s and 1990s emerged from such a closed process as that which generated the internal market reforms. In the field of primary care, for example, the government issued a Green Paper outlining its proposals. Following consultation with the professions, the government dropped some of the more controversial proposals (for example, a plan to introduce health care 'shops' which would allow outside organisations to provide integrated primary care services – an idea which has since resurfaced on a number of occasions). Nevertheless, the intention to link the remuneration of primary care professions to their performance, a key theme of the government's proposals, was pursued with some vigour. In the case of the GPs, negotiations over a new contract subsequently broke down and a new settlement was imposed, without further consultation.

Compared with its predecessor, the Major government (1990–97) placed a greater emphasis on consultation on new health policy initiatives. The Health of the Nation strategy, for example, began as a Green Paper, and following consultations, a White Paper emerged setting out the government's plans. It also showed a greater willingness to issue proposals in draft form, with amendments being made after a period of consultation. An example was the Code of Practice on Openness in the NHS, which was modified considerably following heavy criticism of an earlier draft. A move in the direction of a more open system of consultation was indicated in 1995 when the Department of Health embarked on a 'listening exercise' as part of its plans to review the future of primary care. The results of this consultation exercise were subsequently published by the department as a means of encouraging debate about future options.

In spite of these examples, the authoritarian style of decision making that characterised the 1980s persisted to some extent into the following decade. This was particularly evident with regard to policies that appeared to challenge the ethos of the NHS, such as the Private Finance Initiative (which attempted to extend the role of the private sector in the building and operation of NHS facilities) and market testing (an extension of the contracting out scheme introduced in the previous decade).

Legislation

As in many other areas of policy making, the large Commons majorities enjoyed by the Thatcher governments between 1979–90, coupled with the lack of constitutional constraints, created the ideal conditions for radical legislation. The Thatcher government's grip on the Parliamentary process was exemplified by the passage of the NHS and Community Care Act 1990, which provided a statutory basis for the internal market and the community care reforms. Despite the controversy surrounding these reforms the government steered its proposals through Parliament with very few problems. Debate was limited by use of a Parliamentary measure known as the 'guillotine', which ensured that most of the 252 new clauses and amendments added to the bill during its passage were carried without debate.

The government, in the face of opposition from some of its own backbenchers and the House of Lords, made a number of concessions. These included the creation of a Clinical Standards Advisory Group – to report on the impact of the reforms. This and other concessions made during the passage of the bill (such as the extension of the Audit Commission's brief to investigate the impact of ministerial decisions) went a small way towards appeasing those who called for the reforms to be evaluated, but was not a substitute for a system of pilot projects or full independent evaluation as advocated by the professions. With a mixture of minor concessions and pressure from party whips, the government was able to see off the challenges to its internal market and community care legislation in both the Lords and Commons. Indeed the only major defeat was on the community care part of the bill, where a Conservative rebellion forced a government re-think on income support for elderly people in residential care.

Policy evaluation

The Thatcher government was frequently criticised not only for its reluctance to consult on policy, but also for its failure to submit policies to evaluation. It refused to pilot the internal market as the professions had urged, on the grounds that this would delay the reforms. Moreover, it would not provide for an independent evaluation programme (though concessions were made during the passage of the legislation to allow some evaluation of the reforms, see above). The pace of reforms and the lack of evaluation was criticised even by one of the architects of reform, the American economist Alain Enthoven.

A limited amount of monitoring subsequently took place under the Major government. For example, in Scotland, the GP fund-holding scheme was independently evaluated. Subsequently, total fund-holding (where GP budgets cover virtually the whole range of secondary health care) and other variations of the fund-holding scheme have been piloted. Later, there was an indication of a more systematic approach to piloting and evaluation. The Conservatives' White Paper on Primary Care, published in 1996, placed considerable emphasis upon piloting and evaluating new arrangements for contracting general medical and dental services (Cmd 3390, 1996).

However, had piloting and evaluation been undertaken, there was no guarantee that the policy would have changed. For example, the Resource Management Initiative was launched in the 1980s on the basis of an agreement between the medical profession and the government that pilot schemes be fully evaluated prior to an extended programme of reform being introduced. Yet before the evaluation study (which turned out to be quite critical of the scheme) was completed, it was announced that the scheme would be extended to other units, much to the annoyance of the medical profession.

Implementation

The Thatcher governments took advantage of a highly favourable political environment. Strong leadership, combined with a large Commons majority, a supportive mass media (although less so perhaps on health than other issues), and a weak and divided Parliamentary opposition, facilitated the introduction of centrally determined policies, unpopular with the NHS workforce and the public. But in spite of this, the Thatcher governments often faced difficulties in implementing its policies.

Even before the reforms of the late 1980s, the Thatcher governments had faced implementation problems in this field. One such case was contracting out, where health authorities were expected to open up services such as hospital cleaning, laundry and catering to private sector competition. Reluctant health authorities repeatedly found ways of keeping their services 'in house' rather than giving the contracts to the private sector, forcing the government to change the rules on a number of occasions. Another policy which faced problems at the implementation stage was general management. Plans to distinguish policy making from management at the top of the NHS failed when the new chief executive appointed by the government resigned complaining of ministerial interference. Meanwhile the appointment of general managers at all levels within the service was hampered by the lack of available talent. Ministers clearly wanted to appoint outsiders rather than NHS administrators, but this proved difficult given the relatively low salaries compared with the private sector, the short-term contracts on offer, and the relatively unattractive career prospects. This, coupled with a few spectacular failures involving general managers drawn from the private sector, led the government to accept that the vast majority of general managers (over four-fifths) would after all come from the ranks of the NHS administrators.

The dilution of the internal market reforms further illustrates the difficulties faced by those implementing policy. There were two main reasons why this policy began to change at the implementation stage. First of all, ministers became alarmed at the electoral impact of the reforms, prompted by a series of by-election defeats where health was a prominent issue. Thatcher herself had doubts about the proposed changes and considered postponing implementation until after the forthcoming general election which could be held no later than 1992 (Thatcher 1993, Timmins 1995). A decision was eventually made to proceed with the health reforms, but to postpone the community care changes until 1993 (largely because of the impact of the new regime on community charge bills prior to the election).

There were also practical reasons for the slowdown. The NHS, as many observers had warned, was simply not in a position to implement the policy. The infrastructure of the new internal market – staff, computers, financial systems, could not be put in place in so short a space of time. The most serious problem was the lack of information about costs and activity – essential if the contracting process was to operate as originally envisaged.

Changes to the internal market policy continued following Thatcher's departure. Major faced a far less favourable political environment than Thatcher, presiding over an increasingly disunited government, a divided party, a hostile media, and an effective Parliamentary opposition. After 1992, the circumstances became even more difficult as the government's majority began to shrink, as a result of by-election defeats and defections, and eventually, disappeared. But before this, the policy had already begun to shift, with the Department of Health calling on health authorities and trusts to adopt a 'no surprises' approach, so that the new contracts would not disturb existing patterns of provision. A number of other moves reinforced the steady state, including the postponement of a population-based funding formula (which protected to some extent areas that would lose resources under the new regime), and the temporary withdrawal of the London hospitals from the internal market.

Following the 1992 general election, the Conservative government continued to alter its policy, often making changes in response to outside pressure from the media and organised interests. For example, a series of financial scandals in the NHS amid a broader public concern about 'sleaze' in public life, led to the introduction of Codes of Openness, and Codes of Conduct and Accountability for health authority members. Complaints from within the NHS about the absence of a clear framework for intervening in the market, and wider concerns about the efficacy of market forces led to the production of regulatory guidelines in 1994. In the following year, the government responded to complaints about the lack of accountability of GP fund-holders by introducing a new framework of planning and accountability. Furthermore, in view of the pressure on government to cut back on the bureaucracy stimulated by the market and other reform initiatives, the government rationalised the structure of the NHS in 1996 (abolishing the Regional Health Authorities and merging District Health Authorities and Family Health Service Authorities) and embarked upon a drive to cut management costs.

Although the Major government drifted from the more explicit market approach initially advocated by its predecessor, its openness and responsiveness to outside pressures should not be overexaggerated. First, although prior consultation on policy improved, there were still shortcomings, the government adopting an authoritarian approach on issues such as the private finance initiative. Second, many of the changes were as much a response to the belligerent right wing of the Conservative party, which believed the internal market reforms had failed to live up to the ideals they promoted, as concessions to outside pressure. The right wing of the party supported measures such as the rationalisation of the NHS structure and management cuts while denying that the market was responsible for the growth in bureaucracy, duplication and inefficiency.

The Conservative government's approach was tempered with pragmatism, particularly at the implementation stage of policy making during the 1990s. In addition its authoritarian style of policy making became slightly more open and responsive as policy was implemented and reviewed. There were three main reasons why this happened. First, changes of personnel were important. Major was more convincing in declaring his support for the NHS than his predecessor had ever been. In addition, the ministers in charge of the Department of Health from 1990 onwards were acknowledged as having a far more conciliatory style than Kenneth Clarke, who as Secretary of State for Health in the Thatcher Government had antagonised the professions and other organised interests during the NHS review and subsequent legislation. Second, the internal market reforms, rather than taking the NHS off the political agenda, fuelled the debate about underfunding, inequitable access to health services, and other problems in the NHS. In 1994 a memorandum leaked from Conservative Central Office revealed the government's concerns, acknowledging continued public hostility to the NHS reforms and calling for 'zero media coverage of the NHS'. But this concern also led the government into a search for practical and workable solutions that involved those directly affected by policy. Third, and related to this, the emergence of technical problems at the implementation stage, revealing flaws that often had been foreseen earlier by others, forced the government to seek the co-operation of professionals and their representatives. This re-opened channels of communication that had been damaged during the late 1980s and indicated a movement towards a more incremental and consensual approach to reform.

A moving consensus?

The Conservative government developed and implemented policy ideas generated by its opponents. By the same token, political adversaries also came round to accept key parts of the Conservatives' health policy agenda. For example, general management was opposed by Labour at the time of its introduction in the mid-1980s. Yet once the new management structures were entrenched, the party decided against reversing the reforms. Similarly, both the Labour Party and the Liberal Democrats came to accept the principle of the purchaser-provider split in the NHS, which the Conservatives had introduced.

However, both opposition parties sought to distinguish their approach from the market-oriented reforms of the Conservatives by emphasising the need for structures which encouraged collaboration and strengthened accountability. They also called for greater regulation to ensure that competition did not undermine the efficiency and quality of health services. Yet, as noted, Conservative policy had already begun to move in this direction.

The health policy documents issued by the opposition parties during the mid-1990s revealed the extent to which they had begun to accept key aspects of the Conservatives' reforms. The Liberal Democrats acknowledged that 'those who propose the reversal of all the recent NHS reforms are living in the past' (Liberal Democrats 1995: 8). A Labour Party document of the same year stated that ' it is clear that it is neither possible nor desirable to turn the clock back. Nor is there any appetite in the health service for huge upheaval. We do not intend to replace one dogmatic approach with another.'(Labour Party 1995: 3).

The Labour and Liberal Democrat parties increasingly accepted the importance of key issues raised by the Conservatives during their years in office. Namely, public expenditure restraint, improving 'value for money', encouraging voluntarism and self-help, seeking out alternative sources of finance, the development of new managerialist techniques and the extension of consumer choice. Operating within this constraint, the Liberal Democrats and the Labour Party were reluctant to commit much in the way of additional public resources to health care, and conceded that there were limits to state care accepting, for example, a larger role for the voluntary sector. These parties also focused much more on the improvement of efficiency and quality of service, and placed greater emphasis on the role of the health care consumer than pre-viously.

How can the vitriolic debates over health care reform be squared with the gradual convergence of policies? One explanation is that there is a moving consensus, as described earlier by Rose and Davies (1995), in health care. Despite the hostility between the government and the opposition parties on health care issues, certain factors have led policies to converge.

Governments, both in office and 'in waiting', are constrained by a range of factors which encourage policy convergence and continuity. Political limits are imposed by the social context. Public opinion, the media and pressure groups, can restrict the options available to the parties and influence decisions during the policy process. These political pressures are evident particularly at the implementation stage of health reform. Such pressures have had an impact on opposition parties too. Notably, in opposition both the Labour Party and the Liberal Democrats sought to incorporate outside views before publishing their definitive policy documents.

Opposition parties' policies during the 1980s and the early 1990s were shaped by two political perceptions. First, that many within the NHS opposed further radical reform. This pushed the Labour and Liberal Democrat parties in the direction of incremental, piecemeal reform rather than a 'big bang' approach. Second, it was clear that groups and indivi-duals that had benefited from the reforms would vigorously oppose plans which threatened such gains. For example, Labour's plans to abolish GP fund-holding were heavily criticised by the director of the National Association of Fund-holding Practices, who warned that this could lead to protests from fund-holding GPs, and ultimately to their exodus from the NHS. Similarly policies inimical to private health care would be opposed by a much stronger lobby, in view of the growth of this sector.

The opposition parties also realised that public opinion could not necessarily be relied on to support a reversal of the reforms. Indeed, as the reforms became part of the landscape, significant elements of public opinion could conceivably be mobilised against such moves. By 1996 GP fund-holding covered over half the population in England and Wales. Reversing this policy was therefore likely to be controversial, particularly as fund-holders actively began to seek public support for the scheme. In the case of private health care, similar considerations applied. Although only a minority of people (around one in eight of the population) had private health insurance, and many of these used the NHS as well as the private sector, any policy aimed at discouraging private care would offend a much larger proportion of the public than would have been the case in 1979.

Potential technical problems associated with future reform also shaped the policies of the opposition parties. As the new structures and processes introduced into the NHS became entrenched, the costs of reversing the health reforms were increasingly perceived as prohibitive, both in terms of financial costs and opportunity costs (for example, legislative time involved in introducing new statutes). Moreover, the Labour Party and the Liberal Democrats began to accept that, at least in the short-term, it would be impossible to reverse certain structural and procedural changes, such as mergers between health authorities and between trusts, contracting processes which determine patient flows, and joint working arrangements between the NHS and the private sector.

Finally, significant shifts within the dominant opposition party further reduced the prospects that the Conservatives' reforms would be reversed. The Labour Party underwent a considerable shift in its stated values in the first half of the 1990s. Though this initially had little impact on its health policy, some within Labour Party circles began to question whether collective provision was after all the best way of delivering efficient and equitable health care. As a result greater support arose for the non-state sector in the financing and provision of care. There was also a greater emphasis on quality of service and the user's perspective, and endorsement of the contract culture of welfare introduced by the Conservatives (see Abel-Smith & Glennerster 1995, Mandelson & Liddell 1996).

While the opposition parties came to accept part of the government's reform agenda, the governing party too was influenced by past policies and the agendas of its opponents, as we saw earlier. Competition between the opposition and the governing party is not therefore a one-way street. However, governments are keen to emphasise differences between its policies and those of the opposition, and rarely acknowledge that they have been influenced by their opponents. By the same token, opposition parties are reluctant to give any credit to the government's reform programme.

Conclusions

The party rhetoric which pervades the adversary system of British government and politics exaggerates the appearance of disagreement between the main parties. This makes it difficult to distinguish real policy differences from ideological and electoral posturing. In recent years, given the heightened political significance of health issues it has become even more difficult to analyse the true extent of disagreement and consensus. These difficulties are compounded by the adoption of a narrow concept of consensus that focuses on short-term policy agreement.

Consensus in the health policy field is a more complex concept relating to the policy process and to longer-term interactions of the major players. Although disputes over policy often have been fierce, there is evidence of a moving consensus in health care. The Conservative governments of Thatcher and Major slowed down, diluted and reformed their radical policies and adapted policies advanced by the opposition. Meanwhile, the Labour and Liberal Democrat parties, recognising the political and practical constraints involved in reversing 18 years of reform, came to accept both the reform agenda set by the Conservatives and key aspects of government policy.

The initially cautious approach of the newly elected Labour Government in its reluctance to criticise the substance of its predecessor's reforms further supports the moving consensus hypothesis. However, the policy process is rarely predictable, and much depends on the wider political environment within which government operates, particularly the size of its majority in the House of Commons and its ability to maintain party discipline. The Blair Government, like the Thatcher Governments of the 1980s, is blessed with a large working majority. It is possible that it may be tempted to embark upon a more ambitious programme of reform at a later date. However, even where a government has such strengths, as we saw in the case of the Thatcher governments, other political and technical factors come into play at later stages in the policy process to constrain and modify radical initiatives.

Postscript

The Blair government's White Paper on NHS reform, published in December 1997, provides a further test of the moving consensus hypothesis (Cm 3087, 1997). Some of the headline proposals – abolition of the internal market and GP fundholding in particular – indicate a reversal of previous policies. The new government also placed a greater emphasis than its predecessor on fairer access to services and tackling health inequalities. However, a closer inspection reveals that in many respects the proposals represent a development rather than a reversal of the previous Government's approach. The White Paper's emphasis on promoting clinical effectiveness and internally-generated resources through improved efficiency are consistent with the previous government's agenda. What seems to be intended is a gradual shift towards a more coherent system of commissioning and providing care at local level, a trend that was already in motion before Labour came to power.

References

Abel-Smith, B. & Glennerster, H. (1995) Labour and the Tory Health Reforms. *Fabian Review*, **107** (3) June, 1–4.

Bosanquet, N. (1994) Improving health. In: *British Social Attitudes: The 11th Report* (eds R. Jowell, J. Curtice, L. Brook, D. Ahrendt & A. Park), pp. 51–60. Dartmouth, Aldershot.

Butler, J. (1992) *Patients, Policies and Politics before and after Working for Patients*. Open University Press, Buckingham.

Cmd. 9663 (1956) *Report of the Committee of Inquiry into the cost of the NHS* (The Guillebaud Report). HMSO, London.

Cmd. 7615 (1979) *The Report of the Royal Commission on the National Health Service*. HMSO, London.

Cmd. 3390 (1996) *Choice and opportunity. Primary are the future*. HMSO, London.

Cmd 3807 (1997) *The New NHS: Modern, Dependable*. The Stationery Office, London.

Fowler, N. (1975) *Hansard* 898, 27 October, Column 1031. HMSO, London.

Green, D.S. (1987) *The New Right: The Counter Revolution in Political, Economic and Social Thought*. Wheatsheaf, Brighton.

Illich, I. (1975) *Limits to Medicine*. Penguin, Harmondsworth.

Ingle, S. & Tether, P. (1981) *Parliament and Health Policy: The Role of MP 1970–5*. Gower, Aldershot.

Kavanagh, D. (1985) 'Whatever happened to consensus politics?' *Political Studies*, **33**, 529–46.

Kennedy, I. (1981) *The Unmasking of Medicine*. Allen & Unwin, London.

Klein, R. (1995) *The New Politics of the NHS*. Longman, London.

Labour Party (1995) *Renewing the NHS: Labour's Agenda for a Healthier Britain*. Labour Party, London.

Liberal Democrats (1995) *Building on the Best of the NHS*. Liberal Democrats, London.

Mandelson, P. & Liddell, R. (1996) *The Blair Revolution: Can New Labour Deliver?* Faber and Faber, London.

Rose, R. & Davies, P. (1995) *Inheritance in Public Policy: Change Without Choice in Britain*. Yale University, New Haven.

Smith, T. (1979) *The Politics of the Corporate Economy*. Martin Robertson, Oxford.

Thatcher, M. (1982) *Speech to the Conservative Party Conference*, Brighton, 8 October.

Thatcher, M. (1993) *The Downing Street Years*. Harper Collins, London.

Timmins, N. (1995) *The Five Giants: A Biography of the Welfare State*. Harper Collins, London.

Webster, C. (1988) *The Health Services since the War*. Vol. I: *Problems of Health Care. The National Health Service before 1957*. HMSO, London.

Webster, C. (1994) 'Conservatives and consensus: the politics of the NHS 1951–64.' In: *The Politics of the Welfare State* (eds A. Oakley & A.S. Williams), pp. 54–74. UCL, London.

Webster, C. (1996) *The Health Services since the War*. Vol. II: *1958–1979*. HMSO, London.

Wistow, G. (1992) 'The National Health Service.' In: *Implementing Thatcherite Policies* (eds D. Marsh & R. Rhodes), pp. 100–16. Open University Press, Buckingham.

Chapter 10
Professionalism and Health Care

Mike Saks

Introduction

This chapter focuses on providing an historical and contemporary overview of professionalism in health care in Britain. The emphasis here is on the analysis of professional groups involved in delivering health care rather than individual professional practitioners in themselves – which, though interrelated, are by no means synonymous areas of study (Saks 1995). The chapter begins by outlining in fairly abstract terms the main theoretical debates surrounding the nature and role of professions in the Anglo-American context. The meaning of the concept of professionalism adopted here is then illustrated through the classic case of medicine, which rose to a powerful position in the occupational pecking order in nineteenth century Britain. The form of the social closure achieved by this profession is contrasted with that obtained by the increasing array of other practising professions in the health care division of labour, whose subsequent emergence under the umbrella of medicine is also charted.

It is argued in this chapter that the growth of the range of allied professional groups, from dentistry through to nursing, shows that the field of professions is not static, but shifts over time as the roles of health care occupations develop and the relationship between them ebbs and flows. This is highlighted by an outline of the recent incipient moves towards the professionalisation of alternative medicine, which also raises the wider question of how far the traditional dominance of the medical profession is being eroded by trends in relation to the professions in Britain, not least in the context of changing government health care policy. The chapter concludes by examining the potential public benefits and drawbacks of professionalism in the health sector – an analysis that inevitably leads to questions about the future relationship of professions with the state.

The nature of a profession: definitions and interpretations

A number of different notions of a profession can be identified in the Anglo-American social scientific literature, where the definition espoused depends very much on the theoretical approach adopted by the enquirer. The taxonomic tradition dominated the study of the professions in health care and other fields in the period up to the 1960s. It was based on the belief that professions both share special features that distinguish them from other occupations and play a positive part in society. The identification of the professions within this tradition took two forms. The first was the trait approach centred on the construction of fairly arbitrary sets of criteria seen to represent the main characteristics of a profession, including such factors as the theoretical content of their training and the existence of ethical codes (see Millerson 1964). The second was the functionalist theory of professions in which the core elements of a profession were limited to those held to be of functional relevance to the social system and/or the relationship between professionals and their clients. On this conception, professional groups were generally viewed as being given their privileged socio-economic position and right to self-regulation in exchange for the non-exploitative control of complex and esoteric knowledge of great importance to society (as exemplified by Goode 1960).

The highly favourable and empirically suspect assumptions about professions that underpinned this interpretation – mirroring the ideology of professional groups themselves – did not generally survive the more critical climate that increasingly emerged in the latter half of the twentieth century. The watershed period of the 1950s and 1960s saw interactionists taking the lead in this respect by defining professions not as a neutral, scientific category, but as a socially negotiated symbol in the politics of work (see, for instance, Hughes 1963). This interpretation in turn, though, was subject to criticism as it focused more on small-scale professional case studies than macro-professional issues and was not always empirically well founded. Defining a profession as an occupation that had simply gained the honorific title of a profession as part of a social process also did not sufficiently explain why success or failure was achieved – or indeed what the substantive implications of success were for occupational groups regarded as being professional in nature.

The neo-Weberian approach to professions, which has since come to dominate the field, however, represents a significant improvement in terms of its conceptualisation of a profession. Central to this approach is the notion of social closure that refers to the process by which occupational groups are able to regulate market conditions in their favour in face of competition from outsiders by limiting access to a restricted group of eligibles, enabling them effectively to monopolise available opportunities. Parkin (1979) distinguishes two main types of social closure which are useful heuristic devices in this context. The first is that of usurpation that is centred on improving the standing of a subordinate group at the expense of a dominant group. The second is that of exclusion, on which professionalisation is based, which is linked with the downward exercise of power through the subordination of socially conceived inferiors. Professions typically gain exclusionary closure by pursuing a credentialist strategy underwritten by state licensure.

It is this more concrete neo-Weberian form of social closure that this chapter will take as pivotal to the study of professionalism in the health field. Importantly, this approach provides a strong framework for considering the socio-political factors that have influenced the attainment of the legally underpinned privileges of professions. It also shares with interactionism the advantage of not making unwarranted assumptions about professions based on the uncritical acceptance of their own ideologies about, among other things, the uniqueness of their esoteric knowledge and altruistic orientation. These advantages are tempered by the fact that, while this perspective has been productively employed, neo-Weberian authors have frequently been lured into making unsupported comments about the negative aspects of professionalism. This should not, however, tarnish the general approach to professionalism, which also encourages a more critical, macro-historical analysis of the development of professionalisation in terms of occupationally based power and interests (Saks 1983).

A number of further points need to be noted, before moving on to the specific discussion of the health arena. The first is that neo-Weberian conceptualisations of the professions vary in the extent to which they are based on the original Weberian concept of closure. At one end of the spectrum, professionalism may be classically viewed as a high status occupational strategy designed to control the market for specific services, involving legally defined, self-governing occupations that impose restrictions on entry (see, for example, Collins 1990). At the other end of the spectrum, conceptions of professions have been put forward by neo-Weberian authors that are more indirectly derived from the market-based notion of social closure – in which they are seen, for instance, as occupations where the producer defines consumer needs and how they are satisfied (Johnson 1972) or forms of employment where autonomy exists over technical judgement and the organisation of work (Freidson 1994).

It should be stressed too that there are other contemporary rivals to the neo-Weberian approach to the professions. Of these a major competitor has been the Marxist interpretation of professions which focuses on the relations of production rather than those of the market. Contributors in this camp have also usually taken a less benevolent view of the professions, which are either wholly or partly associated with the oppressive capitalist class, depending on their function in the wider division of labour (see, for instance, Ehrenreich & Ehrenreich 1979). Their work parallels neo-Weberian writers in tending to make overly sweeping, unsubstantiated statements about the professions. One of the main advantages that the neo-Weberian has over the Marxist approach, though, is its sharper analytical conception of a profession. In this respect, Marxist authors typically define professions vaguely in terms of such descriptive indices as preferential pay and security of employment, often linked unsatisfactorily with self-fulfilling notions of the capitalist state, rather than employing the more incisive concept of social closure (Saks 1983).

The classic case of the medical profession

A discussion of the classic example of the medical profession, which can be seen to be an archetypal profession along with that of the legal profession in Britain, illuminates the application of the neo-Weberian concept of social closure in the health arena. In the three hundred years immediately prior to the mid-nineteenth century in this country there was no national system of legally underwitten exclusionary closure in existence – despite such pockets of legal privilege as that provided by the sixteenth-century charter allowing the Royal College of Physicians to oversee medical practice within seven miles of the City of London. The field in fact was a relatively open one in which a broad span of therapies from herbalism and bonesetting to bleeding and purging were available from all kinds of practitioners in competition with each other in the market-place (Porter 1989). In this situation, the predecessors of the contemporary medical profession – including apothecaries, surgeons and physicians in the process of forging their identities – were in a distinct minority, disunited and without consistent educational standards, even by the first half of the nineteenth century (Porter 1987).

The 1858 Medical Registration Act paved the way for the social closure that has been the defining characteristic of the medical profession in the modern context. This Act, which was only passed after much debate inside and outside Parliament, provided for the legally under-written self-regulation of the newly unified, restrictive medical profession that formally excluded the medically unqualified from its ranks (Waddington 1984). Critical to its self-regulatory powers was the centralised control the profession gained through the General Medical Council over education and training, the register of qualified practitioners and its own internal disciplinary affairs. Associated with this elevated occupational standing came many long-run rewards for insiders, not least being expanding income, status and power. As such, it is not surprising that Parry & Parry (1976) have seen the rise of the British medical profession as a classic case of upward collective occupational mobility linked to the neo-Weberian concept of social closure – especially following the reinforcement of the 1858 Act by further legislation, including the 1886 Medical Act, which more starkly clarified its elevated position.

Even this legislation, however, did not formally outlaw the diminishing number of its unorthodox competitors who in Britain – as distinct from many other European countries – remained free to operate under the Common Law, although they could not claim to be registered medical practitioners (Saks 1992). In this sense, the profession achieved more of a *de facto* than a *de jure* monopoly, which was pivoted on the Medical Registration Act that underwrote the exclusive rights of doctors over state medical employment. This meant that, with the subsequent establishment of the 1911 National Health Service Act and the 1946 National Health Service Act, the medical profession not only gained legally based self-regulation and a claim to state enshrined legitimacy, but also managed to monopolise the market in the rapidly growing public sector. Its position of pre-eminence was further confirmed by legislation in the first half of the twentieth century that restricted the conditions – spanning from cancer and cataracts to diabetes and epilepsy – that non-medically qualified practitioners could claim to treat in the private sector (Larkin 1995).

While this helps to define the distinctive and exclusive form that social closure took in respect of medicine in Britain, it is also worth noting that a range of explanations have been put forward from a neo-Weberian perspective to explain its success in gaining exclusionary standing from the mid-nineteenth century onwards. Johnson (1972), for example, relates the rise of professionalism in medicine to the wider sources of power of doctors and the large and comparatively fragmented source of demand from consumers of health care following the industrial revolution. Berlant (1975) meanwhile places more emphasis on the competitive tactics employed by the medical profession in revising its ideology to head off early liberal attacks on corporate monopolism. Importantly, though, both of these accounts stress the complex socio-political dynamics of the situation, not only avoiding the strait jacket of Marxist interpretations based on the fulfilment of the global functions of capitalism, but also representing a substantial advance on the taxonomic approach which tends reflexively to view the autonomy granted to the medical profession in terms of the functional significance of its knowledge to society (Saks 1983). This latter position is problematic given that the medical monopoly was first obtained when heroic medicine was still widely employed, before the introduction of asepsis and anaesthesia and when hospitals were often viewed by the poor as 'gateways to death' (Waddington 1984).

Whatever the explanation of the exclusionary closure achieved by the medical profession, however, the profession had gone from strength to strength by the twentieth century on the basis of its increasingly biomedical frame of reference. This developed with the move away from 'bedside medicine' linked to the patronage system in the eighteenth century, in which rich clients had substantial control over their diagnosis and treatment. The shift was first towards 'hospital medicine' and later 'laboratory medicine' as the twentieth century unfolded – where the subordination of the patient to the doctor through the focus on the classification of disease was increased by the use of laboratory diagnosis and medical intervention without significant reference to the individual (Jewson 1976). This emphasis on the 'scientific' paradigm of biomedicine, in which the body is conceived as a complex of cells separable into parts that could be repaired through the application of drug and surgical regimes, provided the basis of the esoteric medical knowledge on which the profession came to be founded and on which the health care division of labour expanded in contemporary Britain.

The establishment of other orthodox health professions

This development encompassed many occupational groups commonly regarded as professional – including the growing number of health administrators and managers as well as other orthodox health care practitioners. Of the latter, on which this chapter focuses, the groups which have exhibited the highest degree of legally enshrined closure within the marketplace are dentists, opticians and pharmacists. The 1878 Dentists Act gave the General Medical Council the power to examine and register dentists, with the formation of a Dental Board and subsequently a General Dental Council through legislation in the 1920s and 1950s respectively closing the profession to outsiders (Nettleton 1992).

As such, dentists followed a similar trajectory to ophthalmic opticians who, with early origins in the Royal Charter granted to the Worshipful Company of Spectacle Makers in 1629, established the General Optical Council in 1958 which gave them independent professional standing (Larkin 1983). Pharmacy shared significant roots in the past too, going back to the preparation and sale of medicines by chemists and druggists. From this practice sprung the Pharmacy Acts of the 1850s and 1860s which, among other things, gave the Pharmaceutical Society of Great Britain the statutory right to register pharmaceutical chemists and to prevent the unqualified from dispensing medicines (Levitt *et al.* 1995).

For all this legislation effecting social closure, however, dentists, opticians and pharmacists have nonetheless remained in the shade of medical domination as professional groups because their independence from direct medical supervision has been won at the price of being contained within their own boundaries. In this light, it is not surprising that Turner (1995) has viewed these professions as being based on 'occupational limitation' to a specific part of the body or a particular therapeutic method. He also identifies a further more common form of medical domination as that of 'subordination' in which the activities of health care occupations are formally delegated by the medical profession, with restricted scope for autonomy – as in the case of allied health professional work like medical laboratory sciences and midwifery. This is particularly well illustrated by the professions supplementary to medicine which accept patients only through referral from, and under the control of, medical practitioners in the state sector (Levitt *et al.* 1995). Such subjugated occupational groups were established by legislation in 1960 founding the Council for Professions Supplementary to Medicine with its seven initial Boards for chiropodists, dieticians, medical laboratory technicians, occupational therapists, remedial gymnasts, radiographers and physiotherapists (Larkin 1983).

Similar patterns of legally based subordination, mixed with the benefits of occupational closure in the market-place, have also been apparent in the case of nurses, who constitute the largest professional group in the health care division of labour in Britain. To be sure, the professionalising strategy of nurses certainly improved their collective position, as epitomised by the passing of the 1919 Nursing Registration Act which created the General Nursing Council as the key regulating body for the newly forged profession. However, although this legislation has since been further embellished by, amongst other things, the establishment of the United Kingdom Central Council for Nursing, Midwifery and Health Visiting which took over the registration and disciplinary function of the profession in 1983, the case of nursing reveals that size alone is no guarantee of pre-eminent professional standing, insofar as nurses remain subordinated within the division of labour by virtue of the legal monopoly that the medical profession continues to hold over diagnosis and treatment (Porter 1992).

In this light, it is understandable that nursing and other professions allied to medicine are still frequently referred to as 'semi-professions'. Indeed, from a neo-Weberian perspective, such occupations as nursing have been viewed as examples of 'dual closure'. This is because, having failed to secure full professional closure, they are seen to combine the exclusionary device of credentialism with the usurpationary tactics of organised labour against employers and the state (Parkin 1979), as accentuated by the significant recent rates of union membership among nurses (Bagguley 1992). In this sense, it should be emphasised that the desire to professionalise can and often does involve the subordination of other less powerful occupations in the health care division of labour. This can be illustrated by the way in which nurses have historically delegated 'dirty work' to auxiliaries as part of the professionalising project, as they continue to do today through the newly constructed role of care assistants (Witz 1994). There are parallels here too in the manner in which groups like chiropodists and radiographers have protected their territory – in this instance against foot aides and darkroom technicians respectively – to maintain their position in the professional pecking order (Saks 1987).

Given that the medical profession has traditionally been dominant within the increasingly pluralistic health care division of labour in Britain, a key question is that of how this can be explained. Functionalist commentators like Etzioni (1969) suggest that this is because the professions allied to medicine intrinsically need less expertise and training than the medical profession in a hierarchically organised division of labour. Neo-Weberian accounts, however, tend to emphasise the conflictual and fluid nature of the relationship between health professions, as opposed to the stronger connections of medicine to the ruling class that typically figure in more mechanistic Marxist interpretations (see, for example, Navarro 1986). For neo-Weberians, this relationship is largely the outcome of interest-based 'turf battles' involving the maintenance and/or advancement of occupational position in terms of power, status and income, which may or may not have a gender dimension in a patriarchal society (Saks 1995). The resolution of such struggles is usually seen as being mediated by the state, which in the case of health care has for long been pivoted on a medical–Ministry alliance that has helped to ensure the ascendance of the medical profession in the division of labour (Larkin 1995). Much the same might be said of the outcome of the conflicts of medical orthodoxy with not only limited and subordinated practitioners, but also the excluded realm of alternative medicine against which it too has largely maintained its supremacy to date – notwithstanding recent moves to professionalise this area.

The emerging health care professions: Alternative therapists

From participating in a thriving and relatively open field, the numbers and influence of non-medical practitioners of what became defined as alternative health care in the wake of the 1858 Medical Registration Act had declined markedly by the end of the nineteenth century. This was mainly as a result of the newly disenfranchised position of alternative practitioners and the growing legitimacy of medical orthodoxy (Saks 1992). The increasing marginality of practitioners of therapies such as homoeopathy and herbalism, which were typically excluded from the undergraduate medical curriculum and stigmatised in orthodox medical circles (Saks 1996), continued into the first half of the twentieth century. Although alternative therapists could still legally practice, they lacked support from the state, as highlighted by their previously documented exclusion from the fast developing public health service. This is further exemplified by the rejection of such cases as that made by the osteopaths to gain a foothold in orthodox medicine in the inter-war period, which reinforced the monopolistic position in the market-place of medicine and allied professions (Larkin 1992).

From the 1960s onwards, though, alternative therapies in Britain became more popular, as indicated by rising trends in consumer demand, the number of non-medically qualified alternative therapists and political support for unconventional medicine – including from parliamentary lobbies and, indeed, government itself. This followed the increasing failure of biomedical orthodoxy fully to live up to its promise in terms of efficacy and safety and the growing search by consumers for a more holistic approach to health care, involving the fusion of mind and body. When added to fears about the impact of European harmonisation on the continuing Common Law right of unorthodox therapists to practise (Saks 1994), the novel recent move by a growing band of unorthodox practitioners to professionalise alternative medicine becomes more understandable. There is certainly a recognisable strategic advantage to its exponents in establishing these hitherto marginalised therapies on sounder organisational and educational principles at present, even if this may not always be sought by individual practitioners (Sharma 1995). The impact that non-medically qualified practitioners have made in this field, moreover, underlines the potentially fluid nature of the health care division of labour.

The present new-found desire for professional standing is well illustrated by the creation of the Council for Acupuncture in 1980, which brought together the British Acupuncture Association and Register, the Chung San Acupuncture Society, the International Register of Oriental Medicine, the Register of Traditional Chinese Medicine and the Traditional Acupuncture Society. The subsequent foundation of the British Acupuncture Accreditation Board served to establish among lay acupuncturists more unified standards of education, ethics, discipline and practice (Saks 1995). Other groups of alternative therapists have also striven to increase their coherence as part of the professionalising process, including the Society of Homoeopaths. This body has established a register and code of ethics and is seeking state recognition, not least on the basis of its accreditation of a number of homoeopathic colleges with more substantial educational programmes. Not all groups of alternative practitioners, though, are at a similar stage – as highlighted by reflexology which has thousands of practitioners, but a very diverse range of training schools with short periods of preparation for practice and little agreement on standards (Cant & Sharma 1995).

The efforts of more strongly organised alternative therapies to gain legally underwritten professional credentials, as distinct from the more superficial trappings of professionalism, were unsuccessful up to the late-1980s. This was mainly because the government was seeking an all-embracing approach to the professionalisation of such therapies, at a time when the overarching bodies that had been formed – such as the Institute for Complementary Medicine and the Council for Complementary and Alternative Medicine – were unable to represent the field as a whole (Sharma 1995). The situation changed thereafter, as the government increasingly took the view that judgements should be made about individual therapies on their merits to determine their place in the health sector. This is highlighted by the case of osteopathy which sufficiently overcame its internal divisions and put its educational infrastructure well enough in order for the Osteopaths Act to be passed in the early 1990s, following a private member's bill – marking a watershed in the development of alternative medicine (Standen 1993).

The significance of this Act from the viewpoint of the professionalisation of alternative medicine in neo-Weberian terms is that it places osteopathy under the control of the new General Osteopathic Council and establishes protection of title, a register, and self-regulation, including a prescribed set of ethical and educational standards. In so doing, it parallels legislation previously enacted to underwrite the position of other allied orthodox health care professions, albeit that it provides no entry in its own right to state-based practice. The importance of this more limited form of social closure, however, is amplified by the fact that it was followed in 1994 by the Chiropractic Act, which established a similar basis for registration by chiropractors centred on the formation of a new General Chiropractic Council (Cant & Sharma 1995). This suggests that the floodgates to the further professionalisation of other alternative therapies could be opening. One central question therefore thrown into focus by the professionalisation of unorthodox – and, indeed, an increasing span of orthodox – health care practitioners in recent times is that of how far they seriously challenge the dominance of the medical profession.

The erosion of the dominance of the medical profession?

The current extent of the dominance of the medical profession in the health care division of labour is a contentious issue, which has been widely discussed in the literature on professions on both sides of the Atlantic (Elston 1991). The notion of dominance as employed here is taken primarily to refer to the relational aspects of professionalism in terms of authority over other occupational groups in the health care division of labour. This is part of a much broader debate in which it has been claimed by some Marxist and other contributors that the medical profession is in the process of becoming 'deprofessionalised' or 'proletarianised' (see, for example, McKinlay & Stoeckle 1988). In this respect, the medical profession in Britain certainly no longer has such a powerful position of influence over the state as it did in the inter-war period. In fact, the professions as a whole in this country came under attack by the last Conservative government, as part of the more general policies it adopted on deregulation (Johnson 1993).

This ideological assault on professions as restrictive groups in the market was initially most apparent in the health field in the case of opticians who had their monopoly over the supply of spectacles removed by the 1984 Health Services Act (Levitt *et al.* 1995). The effects of government policies, though, seem on the surface at least to have been greatest for the medical profession. Following the Griffiths reform, which fostered the principles of business management in the National Health Service in the early 1980s, the implementation of the White Paper *Working for Patients* (1989) changed the structural position of the medical profession further within the division of labour by establishing the internal market in the state health sector. This has, in principle, made the actions of doctors more amenable to medical audit and heightened the prospect of the rationalisation of their activities based on value-for-money criteria. When taken in conjunction with *The Patients' Charter*

(1991), which was formally designed to give greater sovereignty to the consumer, these seem to add up to a potent package that lends substance to arguments about deprofessionalisation.

It may have proved possible previously for doctors strategically to contain, through a process of incorporation and subordination, the wide range of potential occupational competitors in fields such as pharmacy, midwifery and physiotherapy even when they professionalised. However, with the apparent erosion of their established position of power, there now seems to be the scope for a more significant challenge to medicine in the division of labour. This is underlined by the growing professionalisation of alternative medicine. Leaving aside the financial threat posed to the increasing number of doctors who now practise unorthodox medicine in the private sector, the holistic philosophy and generic therapeutic claims of many non-conventional therapists conflict with the guiding principles and scope of biomedical orthodoxy itself (Cant & Sharma 1995). Therefore it is not surprising that the medical establishment should have for so long taken such a negative approach to unorthodox medicine, as epitomised by the scathing report on alternative therapies by the British Medical Association (1986) in which such therapies are equated with primitive superstition, in face of rising public and political support for them.

Arguments about the decreasing dominance of the medical profession, though, are by no means watertight. Even the professionalisation of alternative medicine may not be as challenging as first meets the eye. Interestingly, the most recent report of the British Medical Association (1993) now seeks collaboration with 'complementary' therapists and encourages them to become more fully organised. Crucially, however, it supports their professionalisation only on terms that are acceptable to orthodox medicine including, *inter alia*, the addition of biomedical components to their training programmes; the adoption of a referral system with clear medical responsibility for patient management; and the acceptance of a medical-style regulatory model for overseeing standards. This could be seen as part of the familiar incorporationist strategy adopted by the medical establishment to minimise the growing threat posed by occupational rivals in the interests of the profession. Indeed, it has also limited the challenge by fostering the use of unconventional therapies by doctors and allied health professions within an orthodox theoretical framework for a restricted range of conditions (Saks 1994).

This strategy, moreover, appears to have been effective, not least because of the increasing subscription of alternative practitioners to models of professionalism broadly consistent with medical dominance, at a time when their therapies are mainly used by consumers alongside, rather than in opposition to, orthodox treatment (Thomas *et al.* 1991). Yet if trends related to the professionalisation of alternative medicine in Britain have not yet seriously encroached upon the power base of the medical profession, much the same can be said about other contemporary challenges to its pre-eminent position. Even though it can be argued that notions like 'deprofessionalisation' and 'proletarianisation' have been insufficiently well conceptualised to be rigorously empirically scrutinised, it is clear that the available evidence for a decline in medical dominance in Britain has been overstated. In this regard, for example, the introduction of general managers following the Griffiths reform may in practice have actually increased the control of clinicians over resources at the expense of other health professionals, while the consumer still appears to have little direct influence over medical decision making despite the changing language of responsiveness to the marketplace (Elston 1991).

The medical profession, however, cannot simply be treated as a monolithic whole, as is evident from studying the dynamics of the interplay between the many sub-groups it contains based on work roles. This is well illustrated by the long-term supremacy of hospital specialists over general practitioners which is now beginning to be redressed in the internal market. This is because of the spread of fundholding that allows family doctors to exercise choice in purchasing hospital services, thereby diminishing the power and status of hospital consultants (Allsop 1995). This adds weight to the argument that the recent government attack on medicine has led to a reconfiguration of professional roles rather than their demise *per se* – in much the same way that the terms of entry into the state-based National Health Service in 1948 had the paradoxical effect of strengthening to varying degrees the position of these two groups of medical practitioners (Johnson 1993). This shows that the fluidity in the division of labour in health care applies to relationships between not only professions themselves, but also specific occupational sub-groups within single professions. What, though, is the future of professionalism in health care in Britain?

Whither professionalism in health care?

Crucial to this debate is the question of how beneficial, on balance, professionalism is perceived to be to the wider society. Commentators from the previously outlined trait and functionalist approaches to the professions, which were dominant in sociology some thirty or more years ago, highlight the benefits deriving from such unique professional groups that are generally held to serve the public interest.

Within this frame of reference, the specialised knowledge gained from the long periods of training now associated with the medical profession and allied professional groups clearly could be seen to be advantageous from the viewpoint of the patient, particularly as ever more health professions gain graduate status (Levitt *et al.* 1995). So too could the protection offered to the public by practitioners through the ethical codes policed by professional regulatory bodies involved in health care, which often explicitly stress their altruistic commitment (Harris 1989). Indeed, such positive features of professionalism are usually depicted by functionalists as justifying the considerable privileges accrued by professions in a sliding scale running down from the pinnacle of medicine to less well-established groups in the health care division of labour.

Contributors from other more recent mainstream theoretical perspectives in this field, however, typically emphasise the negative side of professionalism. The neo-Weberian approach to professions in particular, as noted earlier, tends to stress the self-interested involvement of such groups in the competitive health care market which may not always operate to the advantage of the public, notwithstanding the professional ideologies concerned. This is seen as being in evidence from the time at which the medical profession first gained its monopoly in mid-nineteenth century Britain on a highly tenuous applied knowledge base. In more recent years, this point is exemplified by the response of health professions to the emerging agenda of interprofessional collaboration which has become increasingly central to public policy, mainly because it offers the prospect of more cost-effective and higher quality care. Despite the potential benefits to the broader public, it has been argued that such collaborative working may have been inhibited at least in part because of the 'tribalism' of the health care professions (Beattie 1995).

This is not the whole story in terms of the more critical perspectives on professions in health care. As has been seen, Marxist writers have been less positively disposed towards professionalism in this area because of the place of medicine and other health professions in the class structure of capitalism. Here, among other things, they have drawn attention to the deleterious influence of financial and industrial capital on their activities and the legitimating role that professions in the health field play in dealing with the alienation, disease and diswelfare generated by life in an advanced capitalist society (Navarro 1986). In a not too dissimilar vein, recent interpreters of Foucault – in articulating relationships between discursive formations and non-discursive domains in the archaeology of knowledge – have claimed that the professionalisation of areas like obstetrics and dentistry is not so much a progressive development, but part of the apparatus of state surveillance and disciplinary control of the wider population (Arney 1982; Nettleton 1992).

This highlights that the manner in which professions are conceived will depend to some degree on the theoretical starting point of the enquirer. It is vital in coming to a judgement about the value of professional groups, however, that there is a constructive interface with the available evidence within the perspective concerned – as is clear from the recent criticisms of structuralist Marxist, and indeed Foucauldian, contributors for failing to expose their arguments to counterfactual claims (Macdonald 1995). This is underlined in the health field by Porter (1996) who argues that current trends in nursing are more compatible with increasing patient satisfaction and autonomy than engaging in sophisticated social control activity. Whatever the balance of advantages and disadvantages of professionalism, though, there can be no doubt about the importance of the relationship between professions and the state to its future in health care. As this chapter has underlined, the state ultimately sanctions the privileges of such occupational groups and their interrelationship in the division of labour. In this sense, its interpretation of the public benefits or otherwise of the form of social closure achieved will be vital to the place of professions in the health care pecking order in the years to come.

Conclusions

Notwithstanding the current legally underwritten place of doctors at the apex of the professional hierarchy, history suggests that just as theoretical orthodoxies for interpreting the professions can shift, so too can the position of such groups in the health care division of labour. The opportunities for change in Britain today can be underlined by the enhanced professionalising impulse of the 'new nursing' associated with developments in the nursing process, nursing career structures and educational reform (Witz 1994). They are also accentuated by the recent review of the Professions Supplementary to Medicine Act at the request of the National Health Service Executive which promises, amongst other things, to divest its constituent groups of the label 'supplementary' in the shift towards a proposed new Council for Health Professions (JM Consulting 1996). While the dominant position of the medical profession looks secure for the moment in the wider health division of labour, therefore, the future is by no means fixed – as new professionalising departures interface with changing government policy in impacting on the established professional structures underpinning health care in this country.

References

Allsop, J. (1995) Shifting spheres of opportunity: the professional powers of general practitioners within the National Health Service. In: *Health Professions and the State in Europe* (eds T. Johnson, G. Larkin & M. Saks). Routledge, London.

Arney, W. (1982) *Power and the Profession of Obstetrics*. University of Chicago Press, Chicago.

Bagguley, P. (1992) Angels in red? Patterns of union membership amongst UK professional nurses. In: *Themes and Perspectives in Nursing* (eds K. Soothill, C. Henry & K. Kendrick). Chapman & Hall, London.

Beattie, A. (1995) War and peace among the health tribes. In: *Interprofessional Relations in Health Care* (eds K. Soothill, L. Mackay & C. Webb). Edward Arnold, London.

Berlant, J.L. (1975) *Profession and Monopoly: A Study of Medicine in the United States and Great Britain*. University of California Press, Berkeley.

British Medical Association (1986) *Report of the Board of Science and Education on Alternative Therapy*. BMA, London.

British Medical Association (1993) *Complementary Medicine: New Approaches to Good Practice*. BMA, London.

Cant, S. & Sharma, U. (1995) *Professionalisation in Complementary Medicine*. Report on a research project funded by the Economic and Social Research Council.

Collins, R. (1990) Market closure and the conflict theory of the professions. In: *Professions in Theory and History: Rethinking the Study of the Professions* (eds M. Burrage & R. Torstendahl). Sage, London.

Ehrenreich, B. & Ehrenreich, J. (1979) The professional-managerial class. In: *Between Labour and Capital* (ed. P. Walker). Harvester Press, Sussex.

Elston, M.A. (1991) The politics of professional power: medicine in a changing health service. In: *The Sociology of the Health Service* (eds J. Gabe, M. Calnan & M. Bury). Routledge, London.

Etzioni, A. (ed.) (1969) *The Semi-professions and their Organization*. Free Press, New York.

Freidson, E. (1994) *Professionalism Reborn: Theory, Prophecy and Policy*. University of Chicago Press, Chicago.

Goode, W. (1960) Encroachment, charlatanism and the emerging profession: psychology, sociology and medicine. *American Sociological Review*, **25**, 902–914.

Harris, N. (1989) *Professional Codes of Conduct in the United Kingdom: A Directory*. Mansell, London.

Hughes, E. (1963) Professions. *Daedalus*, **92**, 655–68.

Jewson, N. (1976) The disappearance of the sick-man from medical cosmology 1770–1870. *Sociology*, **10**, 225–44.

JM Consulting (1996) *The Regulation of Health Professions: Report of a Review of the Professions Supplementary to Medicine Act (1960) with Recommendations for New Legislation*. JM Consulting Ltd, London.

Johnson, T. (1972) *Professions and Power*. Macmillan, London.

Johnson, T. (1993) Expertise and the state. In: *Foucault's New Domains* (eds M. Gane & T. Johnson). Routledge, London.

Larkin, G. (1983) *Occupational Monopoly and Modern Medicine*. Tavistock, London.

Larkin, G. (1992) Orthodox and osteopathic medicine in the inter-war years. In: *Alternative Medicine in Britain* (ed. M. Saks). Clarendon Press, Oxford.

Larkin, G. (1995) State control and the health professions in the United Kingdom. In: *Health Professions and the State in Europe* (eds T. Johnson, G. Larkin & M. Saks). Routledge, London.

Levitt, R., Wall, P. & Appleby, J. (1995) *The Reorganized National Health Service*, 5th edn. Chapman & Hall, London.

Macdonald, K. (1995) *The Sociology of the Professions*. Sage, London.

McKinlay, J. & Stoeckle, J. (1988) Corporatization and the social transformation of doctoring. *International Journal of Health Services*, **18**, 191–205.

Millerson, G. (1964) *The Qualifying Associations*. Routledge & Kegan Paul, London.

Navarro, V. (1986) *Crisis, Health and Medicine: A Social Critique*. Tavistock, London.

Nettleton, S. (1992) *Power, Pain and Dentistry*. Open University Press, Buckingham.

Parkin, F. (1979) *Marxism and Class Theory: A Bourgeois Critique*. Tavistock, London.

Parry, J. & Parry, N. (1976) *The Rise of the Medical Profession*. Croom Helm, London.

The Patients' Charter (1991). HMSO, London.

Porter, R. (1987) *Disease, Medicine and Society in England 1550–1860*. Macmillan, London.

Porter, R. (1989) *Health for Sale: Quackery in England 1660–1850*. Manchester University Press, Manchester.

Porter, S. (1992) The poverty of professionalization: a critical analysis of strategies for the occupational advancement of nursing. *Journal of Advanced Nursing*, **17**, 720–26.

Porter, S. (1996) Contra-Foucault: soldiers, nurses and power. *Sociology*, **30**, 59–78.

Saks, M. (1983) Removing the blinkers? A critique of recent contributions to the sociology of professions. *Sociological Review*, **31**, 1–21.

Saks, M. (1987) The politics of health care. In: *Politics and Policy-making in Britain* (ed. L. Robins). Longman, London.

Saks, M. (1992) Introduction. In: *Alternative Medicine in Britain* (ed. M. Saks). Clarendon Press, Oxford.

Saks, M. (1994) The alternatives to medicine. In: *Challenging Medicine* (eds J. Gabe, D. Kelleher & G. Williams). Routledge, London.

Saks, M. (1995) *Professions and the Public Interest: Medical Power, Altruism and Alternative Medicine*. Routledge, London.

Saks, M. (1996) From quackery to complementary medicine: the shifting boundaries between orthodox and unorthodox medical knowledge. In: *Complementary and Alternative Medicines: Knowledge in Practice* (eds. S. Cant & U. Sharma). Free Association Books, London.

Sharma, U. (1995) *Complementary Medicine Today: Practitioners and Patients*, revised edn. Routledge, London.

Standen, C.S. (1993) The implications of the Osteopaths Act. *Complementary Therapies in Medicine*, **1**, 208–210.

Thomas, K., Carr, J., Westlake, L. & Williams, B. (1991) Use of non-orthodox and conventional health care in Great Britain. *British Medical Journal*, **302**, 207–210.

Turner, B. (1995) *Medical Power and Social Knowledge*, 2nd edn. Sage, London.

Waddington, I. (1984) *The Medical Profession and the Industrial Revolution*. Gill & Macmillan, London.

Witz, A. (1994) The challenge of nursing. In: *Challenging Medicine* (eds J. Gabe, D. Kelleher & G. Williams). Routledge, London.

Working for Patients (1989). HMSO, London.

Chapter 11
Palliative Care for All?

David Field

Introduction

The twentieth century has seen a vast transformation in the care of people who are dying. In particular, in advanced industrial societies such care is now seen to be largely the province of the medical and nursing professions. The aim of this chapter is to examine the changing nature of the care of dying people in the UK during the second half of this century, locating the 'medicalisation' of dying in its social context. It begins by looking at the transformation of patterns of death and dying in modern Britain and then summarises the sociological research into the care of people who were dying in hospitals during the 1960s and 1970s. The emergence of the modern hospice movement in response to the perceived deficiencies of such care is briefly considered next. The chapter concludes with a critical look at the current concern to extend palliative care services beyond cancer patients to include all people with long-term terminal conditions[1].

Death and dying in modern Britain

During the present century as the medical capacity to treat disease has greatly expanded, experiences such as pregnancy, childbirth and dying, which were once seen as a normal part of life, have been increasingly brought under the scrutiny and control of the medical profession. While the 'medicalisation' of dying has been central to the transformation of how people who are dying are cared for in contemporary Britain it is itself linked to a number of changes in modern industrial societies. Four features in particular can be identified:

- changing population structure
- changes in families and households
- the 'institutionalisation' of dying
- death and secularisation.

Changing population structure

Over the course of this century Britain has seen a substantial increase in the expectation of life at birth and, like other advanced industrial societies, is now characterised by an ageing population. Death rates have been declining and life expectancy has been increasing for over a century, with the reduction in infant mortality rates being particularly marked. In 1850 less than 5% of the population was aged over 65, whereas in 1994 16% of the British population were aged 65 or over. This is projected to increase to 19% by 2021. In 1996 expectancy of life at birth was 74.4 for males (45.5 in 1901) and 79.7 for females (49 in 1901). The survival of the very old continues to improve, with 2.3 million people above the age of 80 in 1994, more than double the number of people over this age in 1961 (Social Trends 1996).

Strongly related to these changes in the population has been a shift in the nature and pattern of disease. Acute infectious diseases have been largely superseded by long-term chronic conditions as the major sources of illness in the society and rarely have fatal outcomes (Table 11.1). In contemporary Britain the main causes of death are chronic and degenerative diseases of the circulatory and respiratory systems and cancers. These are conditions which primarily affect middle-aged and older adults, where death may be expected and where dying may occur over a period of months or years. Sudden and unexpected deaths are unusual. Among young people most are caused by accidents while for older people heart attacks and strokes are the main sources of sudden death.

Table 11.1 Selected causes of death, England and Wales 1993.

Neoplasms	142 446	(25%)
Circulatory diseases	258 156	(45%)
Respiratory diseases	90 870	(16%)
Accidents*	16 843	(3%)
Suicide and self-inflicted harm	3 952	(<1%)
Infectious diseases+	3 781	(<1%)
All causes	578 170	(100%)

Source: Central Statistical Office, *Annual Abstract of Statistics 1996.*
* 1992.
+ includes HIV/AIDS deaths.

Two important consequences of this changed pattern are that chronic degenerative diseases have become major aspects of health care and that the age at which people normally die has been pushed back to well beyond normal retirement age. For example, Seale and Cartwright (1994: 18) report that in two large national studies conducted in 1969 and 1987 the proportion of deaths occurring at the age of 75 or more rose from 40% to 54%. Whereas formerly people would experience a number of deaths among those they were closely associated with, in the present era children rarely experience the death of a close friend or family member and even for adolescents and adults such deaths are uncommon events.

Changes in families and households

Changes in family and household structures (Social Trends 1996) have raised questions about the ability of modern families to meet their responsibilities of care. Since the 1970s the total number of marriages has declined steadily and in 1993 was lower than a hundred years earlier – despite a larger population. The rate of divorce increased nearly sevenfold between 1961 and 1993 and in 1993 was the highest in the European Community. The proportion of remarriages as a percentage of all marriages had increased to 40%. In the 1990s cohabitation was common, with over one-fifth of men and women between the ages 18–49 cohabiting in 1994–95. Household sizes have become smaller, with an increase in one person households from 11% in 1961 to 27% in 1994–95 and a decline in one family households from 74% to 56% in the same period. Although the extended family has by no means disappeared there has been a move to smaller families often living away from their families of origin. By the 1960s three-quarters of married women had two or less children and in the 1990s birth rates were slightly lower. The smaller size of families, the deferral of child-bearing to later in a woman's life, and the increasing involvement of women in paid employment have lead to a progressive reduction in the *availability* of family members to act as unpaid carers for those with a long-term chronic or terminal illness. Further, the fragmentation and complexity of modern family relationships resulting from increased levels of divorce, remarriage and cohabitation have blurred the *responsibilities* for care. For example, who should look after a terminally ill step-grandparent if their own daughter or son is not available? Thus there may be difficulties about both the responsibility of family members for caring for those who are dying and about the availability of family members to undertake such care. Although the move towards institutional care of dying people in modern Britain antedates the dramatic changes in family and household structures which have occurred since 1970, these changes may have contributed to the increase in the proportion of people dying in nursing and residential homes for the elderly and a decline in home deaths, even though the preferred place of death for most people is still the domestic home (Hinton 1994, Townsend *et al.* 1990).

The institutionalisation of dying

At the start of the twentieth century most deaths in Britain occurred in domestic homes but by mid-century over half of all deaths were elsewhere. From the 1970s approximately a quarter of all deaths occurred in the person's own home, with nearly three-quarters occurring in institutions. Table 11.2 presents the most recently available figures. Of particular interest is the decline in hospital deaths (58% in 1984) and the increase in deaths in communal establishments (mainly residential and nursing homes for the elderly) during the late 1980s and through the 1990s. Seale and Cartwright (1994:130) report an increase in the proportion of such deaths from 5% in 1969 to 14% in 1987 and rates of 16% have been reported at the local level. These changes partly reflect the increased emphasis upon the use of general hospitals for acute care and short stays following the 1990 reforms of the NHS. The increase in the proportion of people dying in communal institutions, especially of elderly women, also reflects the ageing UK population and the breakdown of familial support. Unfortunately there is little research evidence about the care of dying people in these settings (but see Field & James 1993, Shemmings 1996).

One of the important consequences of the changing patterns of dying and the place of death, especially the predominance of hospital care, has been the 'medicalisation' of dying, most obviously seen in the greater amount of medical intervention into the process of dying. Illich (1990),

Table 11.2　Place of death, England and Wales, 1992.

Place of Death	Male	Female	All
NHS	56%	53%	54.5%
Communal establishments*	13%	25%	18.5%
Own home	25%	19%	22%
Other	5%	3%	4%
Number of deaths	271 732	286 581	558 313

Source: Mortality Statistics, General: Review of the Registrar General on death in England and Wales 1992, Table 7. Office of Population Census and Surveys (1994). HMSO, London.

* Includes hospice deaths, which account for approximately 4% of all deaths. Percentages do not sum to 100 due to rounding.

claims that not only are there directly negative consequences from medical intervention (e.g. the 'side effects' of drug treatments for cancer) but that reliance on medical expertise diminishes the competence and autonomy of the lay public, excludes other possible sources of help and creates dependency upon the medical profession. As most people die while being treated in hospitals, death is seen more as a failure of treatment than as an inevitable part of life and so people find it more difficult to accept and come to terms with this. Other writers have also suggested that the institutionalisation of death and its 'sequestration' away from society in medical institutions has had a range of negative consequences, especially in terms of attitudes towards death and dying and the ability of people to come to terms with these (Blauner 1966, Mellor & Shilling 1993).

An associated feature of the institutionalisation and medicalisation of death is that death (and when a person can be said to be dying) has become more ambiguous and harder to establish. Indeed, the use of medical technology allows death to be delayed, reversed or suspended in many cases. Sudnow (1967: 74), suggested that: 'a tentative distinction can be made between "clinical death": the appearance of "death signs" upon physical examination; "biological death": the cessation of cellular activity; and a third category, "social death" which, within the hospital setting, is marked by that point at which the patient is treated essentially as a corpse, though perhaps still "clinically" and "biologically" alive'. These distinctions are still valid in the 1990s, (with 'clinical death' usually being defined in terms of 'brain stem' death).

Secularisation

A final factor is the secularisation of everyday life. Setting aside the question of whether or not a person believes in God or the type of higher being they believe in, one of the main functions of religion has been to make sense of death and its place in life. In modern Britain, despite two-thirds of the population claiming some religious affiliation less than 10% of the population claim to be to be 'extremely' or 'very' religious and only 10% attend a religious meeting at least once a week. Further, public confidence in churches is low (Jowell et al. 1992). However, this lack of participation in formal religious activities does not necessarily mean a lack of religious belief and most funerals and cremations in contemporary Britain have some religious input. However, the centrality and influence of religion is noticeably reduced compared to earlier centuries with the result that one important source for making sense of death is no longer available to many people. This has also meant that people may now look to doctors, counsellors and other professionals for the social and emotional support previously sought from religious functionaries.

Some writers have suggested that, as a consequence of secularisation and associated changes to modern societies, there are few of the collective family and community rituals which in previous eras made sense of death and supported the bereaved (Aries 1983, Elias 1985, Gorer 1965). Thus, when they are faced with their own death or that of someone close to them, people may have to come to terms with this without the help of clear collective rules, and with little support from the wider community. It is argued that death, dying and grieving have become highly individualised and that they are viewed with apprehension and fear by most members of our society. Gorer (1965) went so far as to argue that in modern Britain death had become the new taboo which could not be talked about. Such an extreme view is challenged by Walter (1994) who argues that the issues are more to do with the hidden or seque-strated nature of the place of death and the lack of adequate language to talk about death and dying. Drawing attention to the extensive and ever-present mass media coverage of death, he uses the metaphor of religious revival to argue that far from death and dying being taboo subjects in our society there has in fact been a 'revival of death'. This 'revival' is a product of 'post-modern' individualism and is being shaped by the actions of individuals as they seek to choose a 'good death', albeit with the help (or hindrance) of doctors, nurses and other professionals.

A study of older Aberdonians (Williams 1990) provides more sub-stantial evidence about the complexity of lay attitudes and reasoning about death and dying. Williams suggests that different 'strata' of atti-tudes are evident, describing four patterns which people drew upon in thinking about dying and death. 'Ritual death' included the belief that the dying person should be prepared for their death, have had the oppor-tunity to make farewells to their relatives and friends, and be aware they were dying. This is very similar to the pattern Aries (1983) and Elias (1985) suggest existed earlier in European history. While this pattern was strongly evident, the most common pattern was that of 'disregarded death'. This included a preference for quick and unaware dying – although this way of dying was often seen as difficult to cope with for those who were bereaved. A third pattern seemed to be transitional between these two. Finally, there was an emerging pattern of 'controlled dying' focusing around the core ideas of an aware terminally ill person who might wish to have the option of euthanasia. Attitudes were not necessarily clear cut, and people often held what they recognised were conflicting attitudes, e.g. that a quick death was desirable and that death should occur after 'reunion' with their family. Generally speaking the Aberdeen study supports the view that people do not wish to know about their impending death, but does not support the view that death is highly feared. While dying and death may not be especially feared in modern Britain it may be that certain diseases such as cancer or AIDS are particularly feared and that these epitomise more general and unclearly articulated apprehensions about dying and death (Sontag 1979).

Dying in hospitals

Sociological studies in Britain and the USA described the poor quality of terminal care in hospitals in the 1960s and 1970s (e.g. Glaser & Strauss 1965, McIntosh 1977, Sudnow 1967). What emerged very clearly from these studies was the way in which the social organisation of terminal care work in hospitals resulted in the social isolation of those who were dying. In part this reflected general patterns of medical and nursing work in hospitals whose main roles were seen as essentially curative or restorative. In part it also reflected particular practices with respect to patients who were dying. The diverse range of administrative, 'house-keeping', clinical and support activities in hospitals are, of necessity, bureaucratically organised and co-ordinated. Patients had little, if any, control over the resulting routines of hospital life which to a large extent structured their experience. In the 1960s and 1970s, the hierarchical organisation of nursing and the common practice of structuring nursing work by allocating tasks to nurses (e.g. giving bed baths, drug rounds) served to fragment care and to result in more impersonal care than where nurses are allocated to individual patients and are responsible for all their care – the organisation of nursing work which developed during the 1980s. The dominance of medical staff exerted an important influ-ence on the widely accepted view that the patient's duty was to comply with whatever staff required of them in the central task of symptom management. Another general feature of hospital care at this time was poor communication between health workers about the management of the care they were delivering (a feature which persists in many British hospitals). In particular, where there were no well-established pro-cedures between doctors and nurses for dealing with 'breaking bad news' this created difficulties for both nurses and patients. A common research finding was that although patients were satisfied with their physical care in hospitals, they were dissatisfied about the information they received about their care from staff.

Given the emphasis upon intervention and cure and the prevailing medical ethos in hospitals which saw death as the ultimate failure, it is perhaps not surprising that doctors felt compelled to try every possible means to continue life even when the quality of that life was palpably bad, when the patient did not wish to continue living in pain and distress, and when death could only at best be briefly postponed. The main impetus to this misuse of medical and nursing effort seemed to lie in the inability of doctors to admit that they could not 'save' their patients. A contributing factor here appears to have been the failure of many doctors and nurses to come to terms with their own fears and apprehensions about death. These failures of physical treatment combined with the general practice of limiting information given to patients and the poor communication between doctors and nurses to produce what Glaser & Strauss (1965) described as 'closed awareness' contexts, where staff withheld information about their terminal prognosis from dying patients. This led staff and others to withdraw increasingly from social contact with the person once a terminal prognosis had been established. In one of the most graphic studies of the period, Sudnow (1967) described the 'social death' of dying patients in the hospitals he studied as staff (and relatives) progressively came to treat them as if they were already dead. Given these various deficiencies in the practice of terminal care it is hardly surprising that it was seen as unrewarding by those who were supposed to be delivering it, and that it generated high levels of staff stress and distress among patients and their relatives.

As noted elsewhere (Field 1996), the most striking aspect about the care of dying people during the 1960s and 1970s was the widespread practice of attempting to keep them in a state of ignorance about their terminal prognosis. As such attempts usually failed, the patient's isolation was compounded by feelings of anxiety, mistrust and abandonment. There were a number of reasons for this policy of not communicating the news of a terminal prognosis to the patient. Not only was there anxiety about and avoidance of the possibility of a terminal prognosis among doctors and nurses during this period, but there was often genuine uncertainty about outcome, especially about the likely timing of death. It was thought that not revealing a terminal prognosis would protect patients from depression and other negative psychological consequences. Non-disclosure also meant that doctors and nurses did not have to become involved in discussions about dying with patients, thus avoiding disruption of normal work routines. It might similarly 'protect' relatives from involvement in such potentially distressing and uncomfortable discussions. Glaser & Strauss (1965) found that even when 'closed awareness' broke down it was frequently replaced by mutual pretence where everyone pretended that things were 'as usual' but did not explicitly acknowledge that the patient was dying..

Terminal care in British hospitals has changed since the 1960s and 1970s. The development of more effective and reliable control of pain and other physical symptoms, and the wide dissemination of information about and training in these, has enabled better symptom control and palliation. There is also a better appreciation of the interrelations between physical, psychological, and social factors in the management and care of people who are dying. There has also been a shift from 'closed' to 'open' patterns of communication with dying patients about their prognosis and it is widely accepted that the knowledge which staff, the patient and relatives have about the terminal prognosis is a critical dimension in the care of people who are dying. In the 1990s most terminally ill patients – particularly cancer patients – do learn of their prognosis, usually when they are in hospital (Hinton 1994, Seale & Cartwright 1994: 43) although general practitioners, community nurses and others may have to 'unpack' the news and discuss its meaning further with patients and their families.

Perhaps the most important change in the care of people who are dying has been attitudinal. In the 1990s doctors and nurses are more likely to believe that they can offer something to people with a terminal illness. In the 1960s and 1970s it was hard to be positive because medicine, and to a lesser extent nursing, seemed to have so little to offer by way of symptom control or psychological support. In the 1990s as compared to the 1970s there is a greater probability of terminal care which attends to the person and their feelings – rather than merely to their physical symptoms – and a shift from concealment to openness in communications between doctors and nurses and the patients they are caring for. This move toward greater openness and responsiveness seems to reflect the shift within contemporary Britain from a 'collectivist' to an 'individualistic' ethos of choice and responsibility (Field 1996). Nevertheless, practices reminiscent of the 1960s and 1970s can still be found (especially within the nursing and residential home sector), and it is still the case that hospital consultants may forbid nurses to disclose a terminal prognosis, even in the rare cases where a patient asks directly for confirmation of their suspicions that they are dying (Davey 1993). Not all health practitioners are conversant with or sympathetic to the philosophy and practice of palliative care, and the discredited practices of mid-century can still be found in our hospitals and nursing homes while inadequacies and deficiencies in symptom management and communication persist in both hospitals and the community.

Although most people in contemporary Britain die in an institution, it is important to realise that most of their care takes place in their own home, with spouse/partner and family as their main carers. There may be a large amount of interchange between homes, hospitals and hospices during the course of dying and community-based specialist palliative care services are also accessible. Dying in one's own bed in the familiar surroundings of home with family and friends in attendance is still thought to be the best way to die by many people (Hinton 1994, Townsend *et al.* 1990). It has also been suggested that lay carers will cope better with their bereavement if they can take an active part in care, and this is easier to do at home than in a formal institution. However, adequate symptom control and the constant attendance and extra domestic work which such care entails may cause difficulties and although many families wish to look after their relative at home, they may be unable to do so. Further, while they may have spent most of their terminal illness in their home, a number of people do prefer to die elsewhere. Hinton (1994), in a study of cancer patients referred to St Christopher's hospice home care service found a shift away from home towards hospital as the preferred place of death among both those who were dying and their carers as death neared. However, even in the final week before death 54% of those dying and 45% of their carers wanted the death to take place at home.

Hospice care

In modern Britain the hospice movement played an influential part in these changes. From modest beginnings it first became the main alternative to mainstream services for the care of terminally ill cancer patients, and by the 1990s was a recognised and significant partner in the planning and delivery of palliative care services. James & Field (1992) attempted to make sense of the development and change of the modern hospice movement by using Weber's analysis of authority relationships. In its early years the modern hospice movement was led by a few exceptional (charismatic) individuals whose singleness of vision, intensity of purpose and commitment to improving the terminal care of cancer patients motivated their 'followers' and captured the support of the wider public. In particular, the role of Cicely Saunders as a highly visible leader was central to the development of the modern hospice movement in Britain, and also internationally. Another important element was the Christian spiritual calling which inspired and sustained so many of the early hospice workers – both leaders and 'rank and file' workers. The hospice vision of terminal care was in sharp contrast to the hierarchical and medically dominated model reviewed in the previous section. Hospices aimed to provide care by a team of carers in a homely environment which respected and facilitated individual choice and involvement and which was responsive to the physical, social, psychological and spiritual needs of patients and their families. This vision resonated with general fears and apprehension about cancer and dissatisfaction with the impersonal care of people dying in hospitals and other institutions. The hospice philosophy of 'holistic care' whose aim is to maximise the quality of life remaining to those who are dying by palliating their symptoms provides the important ideological under-pinning to present day hospice and palliative care services.

The danger for any charismatic movement is what happens as the movement expands and the original leaders are superseded by their followers. James and Field argue that as the hospice movement developed, the original vision became altered and diluted in various ways by the new recruits to the movement. There were also a number of intra-organisational and external environmental changes, especially in terms of health services, which both challenged and threatened hospice principles. These included increasing bureaucratisation, as hospice organisations began to regularise and stabilise their day-to-day functioning. The increasing requirements for financial and other resources to support and sustain the expanding hospice programmes also contributed to greater formalisation, bureaucratisation and 'professionalisation' of fund-raising and administration. As career paths in hospice care became a reality for health professionals there was also a process of 're-professionalisation' of hospice staff. This, coupled with growing pressures to diversify and expand the range of hospice activities, has led to some competition and strains between different elements within hospices and, more recently, between different specialist palliative care services. Externally, changes within health services such as formal requirements for evaluation and audit of hospice activities and the purchasing of palliative care services on a contractual basis by Health Authorities were also significant in the 'routinisation' of hospice activities.

The emphasis of the hospice movement upon research and the education and training of health workers has been as important, indeed probably more important, in influencing the care of dying people in Britain (and elsewhere) than their actual care of people who were dying. For example, pioneering work on pain control provided both a better understanding of the interaction of physical, psychological and social elements in the dynamics of pain and its better management through the more effective use of drugs. The latter have been easily assimilated into the dominant biomedical approach to treatment but the conceptualisation of 'total pain', although influential, may not have had as much impact upon clinical practice. Hospices also demonstrated that one could talk with terminally ill patients about the fact that they were dying and provided important experience and training for doctors and nurses to do so in an unthreatening and supportive environment. This has been influential in transforming the debate from *whether* to reveal a terminal prognosis to questions about *how* to do so.

Palliative care for all?

The success of the hospice movement in promoting its vision of care which attends to the physical, psychological, social and spiritual needs of the dying person has greatly influenced practice elsewhere and is partly responsible for the development of palliative care as a recognised and important part of health care in Britain and in other countries. Although only a small proportion of people actually die in a hospice (about 4%), in the 1990s hospice and palliative care services include a variety of day care programmes, community nurses and pain and symptom control teams in hospitals. However, fears have been expressed that the development of palliative care, especially the growth of the speciality of palliative medicine, is being accompanied by a process of 're-medicalisation' and the dilution of hospice ideals (Field 1994). There appears to be some substance to these concerns, with increasing numbers of hospices appointing full time medical directors and moving towards more hierarchical authority structures in which some nurse managers are finding their influence and decision-making powers diminished. The concern that the focus of the hospice movement upon dying will come to be replaced with a focus upon symptom management also seems to be confirmed as hospices now perform a greater number and wider range of medical procedures than previously. There is also a considerable momentum within specialist palliative care services (SPCS) to provide palliative care much earlier in the progression of the disease (i.e. further away from the time of expected death) which may also make the focus of care upon dying less central.

The establishment of the National Council for Hospice and Specialist Palliative Care Services in 1992 provided both a forum for the exchange of information and opinions across the range of voluntary and statutory agencies involved in the provision of palliative care and an important vehicle for influencing policy and practice (Gaffin 1996). It also plays an important role in the current drive to extend the scope and practice of palliative care. While this is motivated by a desire to address perceived deficiencies in the care of people who are dying, other factors are also in play. Within the context of a capitalist society it would be unrealistic to imagine that members of hospices and SPCS, despite their altruistic ideology, are immune to the dynamics of organisational expansion, the equation that 'success' is measured by such expansion or to the personal and institutional rewards of exercising power and influence at local and national levels. As the particular interests of organisations and professionals become linked to continuing expansion – e.g. more jobs within SPCS sustains the increasing specialisation and professionalisation of SPCS workers and enhances their possibilities for promotion – there is a danger of 'goal displacement', with expansion being seen as unquestionably good for others because it is what professionals see as good for themselves.

These various factors can be seen clearly in recent calls to extend palliative care services beyond those with cancer. In 1993 the Standing Medical Advisory Committee and the Standing Nursing and Midwifery Committee jointly recommended that all patients needing palliative care services should have access to them, and that services for patients dying from diseases other than cancer should be developed. While most in-patient hospices in Britain have made some provision for people in the terminal stages of motor neurone disease and multiple sclerosis it was not until the advent of AIDS that substantial numbers of non-cancer patients began to receive hospice care, albeit largely in dedicated 'AIDS hospices'. Eve & Smith (1996) estimated that in 1993 only 6% of adult in-patient hospice admissions in the UK and Ireland were for conditions other than cancer, of which HIV/AIDS patients accounted for slightly more than 3%.

The case for extending SPCS to people dying from long-term non-malignant diseases can be made in terms of equity and in terms of need. However, concerns about equity are likely to be insufficient grounds for action – inequalities in health have persisted throughout the history of the NHS yet discussions of them have been conspicuous by their absence from official British government policy documents such as Health of the Nation (1992). In 'post-modern' Britain a more acceptable argument based upon 'moral' grounds is likely to be that which builds upon the increasing emphasis within the society upon the individual. One of the appeals of palliative care may be that it reflects this emphasis as it is premised upon the aware individual exerting choice and control, and upon the right – even the responsibility – of the individual to know their fate. In this view, modern dying, like the rest of modern life, is about control and choice. Extending SPCS beyond cancer patients would extend such choice and control.

A substantial argument for extending SPCS beyond cancer patients can be made on the basis of need. For example, Higginson's review of UK data suggests that high levels of pain and trouble with breathing and significant levels of other distressing symptoms are to be found among patients with 'progressive non-malignant diseases'. Her estimates suggest that among terminally ill patients with such conditions there may be as many people in need of SPCS as can be found among the smaller number of cancer patients (Higginson 1997: 15–17). Addington-Hall's review of studies published in 1966–96 (1998) confirms that significant discomfort and pain may be as (or more) prevalent and severe among terminally ill patients with non-malignant conditions as among terminally ill cancer patients. Such patients were more likely to have worse symptom control, to be dependent upon others for more than six months, to die in a hospital and to die alone. More recent studies awaiting publication substantiate the view that a significant number of people who die from heart disease, strokes and chronic respiratory failure are likely to benefit from SPCS. However, confirming that there is a case for extending SPCS to long-term non-malignant terminal conditions does not guarantee that this will happen. There are at least three potential barriers to achieving such an extension: the costs of extending specialist palliative care services, vested interests in present arrangements and the difficulties of identifying candidates for SPCS.

Costs

While at the local level, Health Authority purchasers are likely to welcome the extension of SPCS in terms of both equity, effectiveness and better integration of services, at the national level the implications of financing such an extension may be crucial. Looking at the three main causes of death in our society suggests that a simple extension of SPCS could at least double the costs of such services (Table 11.1, Higginson 1997). Present SPCS are heavily subsidised and it is questionable whether extended SPCS would continue to be subsidised so heavily by private and voluntary sector contributions. Thus, the wider availability of SPCS would probably require more state funding. Using these crude and simple indices to estimate possible future costs suggests that the increased costs of SPCS could be a formidable barrier to their extension, particularly in a period when the national government is committed to keeping the costs of health services down.

Vested interests

Constraints upon extending SPCS beyond cancer are not simply a matter of how to find the additional costs and other resources to do so. The consequences for other sectors and groups in the health service have also to be considered. The wholesale replacement of existing services by SPCS would be so difficult to implement given the complexity of existing service arrangements, the likelihood of severe disruption to services during the transitional period, and the vested interests already entrenched in the health service, that it is not contemplated. The model is thus one of supplementing and complementing existing services. For example, the National Council for Hospice and SPCS (1997) suggests there will be four models of SPCS provision by the end of the century: an extension of the present community-based hospice system to non-cancer patients; oncology centres; more hospital palliative care teams – which would also cover non-cancer patients; and SPCS for HIV/AIDS patients.

Whatever the model, extending SPCS beyond cancer would require greater integration of SPCS and other 'mainstream' health services. This would threaten vested interests in the present pattern of service delivery, both those in the 'mainstream' health services and also within the SPCS. It would be difficult, for example, for specialist palliative care nurses and physicians to negotiate the appropriate division of labour, patterns of referral, co-operative working and funding of services with hospital-based specialists in cardiac, respiratory and other specialities already dealing with patients who would become eligible for these SPCS. Even if SPCS are simply intended to supplement existing services, they will at least be partly replacing them. With the principle of money 'following' or being attached to patients in the NHS of the 1990s this would have significant consequences for staffing levels, prestige and influence of existing services.

It is a moot point whether hospice services can be extended very much further than at present. The resources of existing hospices are already stretched to cope with terminally ill cancer patients and the small number of mainly neurological patients they admit. It is doubtful whether they could be extended to include other chronic conditions without some sort of rationing and the exclusion of some types of cancer patients currently receiving their services. This may not be acceptable to hospice volunteers and to those who make charitable donations to support their local hospice. If the nature of hospice care changes too much it may lose its support in the community, with possibly severe financial consequences since approximately half the costs of the hospice services are met through voluntary contributions. The possibly negative consequences of extending existing hospice services, especially in-patient services, beyond cancer patients for the integrity and financial viability of local hospice organisations must thus be considered carefully. One solution might be that those concerned to provide palliative care for people with other conditions should follow the hospice example and raise their own money to provide equivalent services. The precedent has already been established with children's hospices (which tend to accept children with all terminal conditions) and HIV/AIDs. However, this would create competition within an increasingly 'tight' and competitive fund-raising environment and does not address the cost implications of substantially extending other SPCS, e.g. hospital support teams.

Given the community based nature of the care for people with long-term chronic and terminal conditions and the emphasis in the late 1990s upon primary care and community based health services, the extension of community based SPCS will be of crucial concern (NCHSPCS 1996). While the present cancer-based SPCS are broadly welcomed by GPs and community nurses there are also some strains between specialist and generalist providers in the community. These might well become worse with the extension of SPCS to patients with chronic diseases, i.e. the patients who provide the bulk of the work for GPs and community nurses. Further, although not a barrier to extending SPCS, it is perhaps worth considering the question of whether in the long run community based SPCS (especially more comprehensive SPCS) may lead to the 'de-skilling' of GPs and community nurses in their care for people who are dying. The extension of SPCS could hasten that process and thus possibly have long-term negative consequences for the care of dying people. There is also the question of tensions within SPCS. Within the current provision of community SPCS there is already some competition and rivalry between existing hospice and other SPCS which are causing strains and local difficulties (e.g. between hospice home care teams and community Macmillan nurses). Further, it is unclear what the effect of extending community SPCS beyond cancer patients might be on their relationships to services such as hospices and other organisations which are restricted to cancer patients (e.g. Macmillan Cancer Relief Fund's charitable status precludes it from extending its activities beyond cancer). Finally, the relationship of extended SPCS to Social Services would also need to be considered. It is likely that similar (but more widespread) problems to those already existing between 'health' and 'social service' agencies would be met in negotiating and deciding responsibility for and funding of the community care of people who are dying.

Identifying candidates

Despite the research suggesting that terminally ill patients with chronic conditions are suitable candidates for SPCS, it seems that doctors find it difficult to identify them in this way (Field 1996). In particular, two important differences between cancer and non-malignant conditions have been suggested: the continuing benefit of conventional restorative treatments and the greater uncertainty about the fact and likely time of death. The latter appears to be the key 'blockage' to extending SPCS because until a patient has been defined as 'terminally ill' they will not be seen by GPs and other health workers as a suitable candidate for palliative care. Whether or not there are 'intrinsic' differences in disease progression is open to debate, but what is not in doubt is that doctors are less likely to see such patients as 'terminally ill' and in need of SPCS. Indeed, many of the issues which characterised the treatment of terminally ill cancer patients in the 1960s and 1970s – adequate pain control, doctor–patient communication and neglect of social and psychological aspects of the illness – are evident when looking at these patients. Even if the various difficulties identified above can be resolved, unless GPs identify chronically ill people as candidates for SPCS it will be very difficult to extend such services to them.

Conclusions

In Britain the care of people who are dying has changed in a number of ways since the 1960s and 1970s. Yet in the 1990s, as in the 1960s, medicine remains centrally involved in providing and defining such care. The hospice movement has greatly influenced such changes in the care of dying people in 'mainstream' health care settings, although the fundamental attitudinal shift towards more 'open' awareness and communication in dealing with dying patients also reflects the greater societal emphasis upon individuals and their rights. However, despite resulting improvements in the care of people who are dying, the good practices of successful palliative care are still patchy rather than uniformly spread throughout contemporary Britain. Such weaknesses and deficiencies are one source of the commitment of hospice and palliative care specialists to expand their influence and services, although inter-professional rivalries and competing definitions of care are also evident. This is evident in the analysis of the social and political issues involved in attempting to extend SPCS to people dying from long-term chronic conditions. Although practical issues concerning resourcing and organising such care must be addressed, central to the success or failure of this endeavour are competing definitions of professionally defined need for a new type of service which, if implemented, would directly affect other elements within the health service. Hence, the power of vested interests in the present system of health care and the extent of resistance of consultants and general practitioners to new patterns of care are likely to prove more fundamental.

Note

1. Terminal care refers to the care of a person whose death is expected within a defined period of time, usually less than a year. Palliative care, while containing the idea that death is likely and certain, refers to the type of care which is provided: care which is concerned to alleviate (palliate) symptoms and to enhance the patient's quality of life. In practice, it is not always easy to differentiate between the two.

References

Addington-Hall, J. (1998) *Palliative Care for Patients with Non-malignant Diseases*. National Council for Hospice and Specialist Palliative Care Services, London.

Aries, P. (1983) *The Hour of our Death*. Penguin, Harmondsworth.

Blauner, R. (1966) Death and social structure. *Psychiatry*, **29**, 378–94.

Cmd 1986 (1992) *The Health of the Nation: A Strategy for Health in England*. HMSO, London.

Davey, B. (1993) The nurse's dilemma: truth-telling or big white lies. In: *Death, Dying and Bereavement* (eds D. Dickenson & M. Johnson), pp. 116–23. Sage, London.

Elias, N. (1985) *The Loneliness of the Dying*. Blackwell, Oxford.

Eve, A. & Smith, A. (1996) Survey of hospice and palliative care inpatient units in the UK and Ireland, 1993. *Palliative Medicine*, **10**, 13–21.

Field, D. (1994) Palliative medicine and the medicalization of death. *European Journal of Cancer Care*, **31**, 58–62.

Field, D. (1996) Awareness and modern dying. *Mortality*, **1** 255–65.

Field, D. & James, N. (1993) Where and how people die. In: *The Future for Palliative Care* (ed. D. Clark). Open University Press, Milton Keynes.

Gaffin, J. (1996) Achievements and intentions – the work of the National Council for Hospice and Specialist Palliative Care Services. *European Journal of Palliative Care*, **3**, 100–104.

Glaser, B.G. & Strauss, A.L. (1965) *Awareness of Dying*. Aldine, Chicago.

Gorer, G. (1965) *Death, Grief and Mourning in Contemporary Britain*. Cresset, London.

Higginson, I. (1997) *Palliative and Terminal Care Health Care Needs Assessment*. Radcliffe Medical Press, Abingdon.

Hinton, J. (1994) Can home care maintain an acceptable quality of life for patients with terminal cancer and their relatives? *Palliative Medicine*, **8**, 183–96.

Illich, I. (1990) *Limits to Medicine*. Penguin, London.

James, N. & Field, D. (1992) The routinization of hospice: charisma and bureaucratisation. *Social Science and Medicine*, **34**, 1363–75.

Jowell, R., Brook, L., Prior, G. & Taylor, B. (eds) (1992) *British Social Attitudes, the 9th Report*. Dartmouth Publications, Aldershot.

McIntosh, J. (1977) *Communication and Awareness in a Cancer Ward*. Croom Helm, London.

Mellor, P.A. & Shilling, C. (1993) Modernity, self-identity and the sequestration of death. *Sociology*, **27**, 411–32.

NCHSPCS (National Council for Hospice and Specialist Palliative Care Services) (1997) *Dilemmas and directions: The Future of Palliative Care*, Occasional Paper 11, London.

Seale, C. & Cartwright, A. (1994) *The Year before Death*. Avebury, Aldershot.

Shemmings, Y. (1996) *Death, Dying and Residential Care*. Avebury, Aldershot.

Social Trends 26 (1996) HMSO, London.

Sontag, S. (1979) *Illness as Metaphor*. Allen Lane, London.

Sudnow, D. (1967) *Passing On: The Social Organisation of Death*. Prentice-Hall, Englewood Cliffs, N.J.

Townsend, J., Frank, A.O. & Fermont, D. (1990) Terminal cancer care and patients' preference for place of death: A prospective study. *British Medical Journal*, **301**, 415–17.

Walter, T. (1994) *The Revival of Death*. Routledge, London.

Williams, R. (1990) *A Protestant Legacy: Attitudes to Death and Illness among Older Aberdonians*. Clarendon Press, Oxford.

Chapter 12
Unwaged Carers and the Provision of Health Care

Veronica James

'No man is an island, entire of it self.

Every man is a piece of the Continent, a part of the main;
If a clod be washed away by the sea, Europe is the less...
Any man's death diminishes me, because I am involved in Mankind:
And therefore never send to know for whom the bell tolls; it tolls for thee.'
John Donne (1627) Devotions

Introduction

Asking students and public service professionals the question 'who are the main contributors to health and welfare remains a worthwhile exercise. In general there is little problem about identifying the NHS and social services, the commercial sector and the charities. The ones that nearly always come last, usually after a considerable amount of prompting, are the informal carers. 'Informal carers' are the millions of people who care for the disabled, the chronically sick, the mentally ill, those with learning difficulties and the elderly, often for many hours a week, for years on end, for no wage. The aim of this chapter is to explore the contribution of these people, questioning why their work has been so poorly understood for so long.

Embedded in the exploration of the work of informal or unwaged carers is a challenging query which most policy-makers dare not ask – the extent to which dependence on unwaged, family carers undermines the life of the carer and the dignity and independence of those being cared for. To offer a response to that query means understanding the range and depth of the significance of unwaged carers; the breadth of their contribution; and the benefits and limitations of users and society being dependent upon them. This generates the further question of whether unwaged carers are able to make the decision to care as purposive human agents, or whether influential social rules and expectations enforce unwaged carers to become part of a structural response, offering them no choice. The first section of the chapter, 'Reading the picture', sets the context of unwaged care, examining the range of terminologies used to describe unwaged carers in order to help establish the accuracy of data on unwaged carers. Next, the numbers and characteristics of unwaged carers are examined together with a resumé of what unwaged carers do and the implications of this work for them. Finally, the contribution of unwaged care is discussed in relationship to the statutory, commercial and voluntary sectors of health care and the contemporary emphasis upon health care in the community.

Reading the picture: terminologies and their tasks

Jimmy, a 16-year-old child carer said:

'When I think about all those years I cared for my dad, it makes me angry, not because I had to care for him – I *wanted* to care for him – but I was left alone to cope with his illness for so long.

'I wasn't just doing ordinary tasks like other kids might do around the house. I was having to cook for him, beg for money and food parcels so I could feed him, take him to the toilet, clean him up when he couldn't get to the toilet – because he couldn't get up the stairs towards the end.

' ...I loved my dad and I couldn't bear to see him losing his dignity – getting more ill before my eyes. But because I loved him, I wanted to be with him. I wanted to look after him. I just wish someone could have helped me and that those who interfered in our lives and made them difficult could have left us alone.'

'...for all those other kids out there who are in the same situation I was, then something should be done to help them. Not take them away from their mum or dad, but to help them care without worrying and being frightened.'

(Aldridge and Becker 1993, Foreword)

Central to this description are two, individual citizens, both in the closed privacy of their shared home and bearing a strain unknown or ignored by helping agencies. Jimmy took on an adult role before he was old enough to vote. The question raised in the introduction is pertinent here. Was Jimmy able to 'choose' this role, or did social pressure 'enforce' his carework for his father?

Yet, in emphasising the work of carers, it is important not to undermine the individuality of those they support. Jimmy's father has been an independent citizen, an individual with adult rights, responsibilities and social standing. It is crucial to understanding the enormity of the work of unwaged carers that the individuality and dignity of each person, as well as the gross numbers of people supported by unwaged carers, be taken into account. In terms of unwaged carer numbers, Jimmy is just one of an estimated 10 000 children under 18 who look after an adult (Aldridge & Becker 1993). Estimations of the numbers of adults involved in this work vary from 1.3 million to 6.8 million depending on definitions of who is included, but despite this structural underpinning of society's health, there are still no agreed terminologies by which to refer those involved.

During the evolution of interconnected systems of commercial, charitable and, increasingly, public health and welfare services during the nineteenth and twentieth centuries, family provision of care remained the norm (Stacey 1988). While family care was complemented by a range of systems to provide for those who had no family, debates about the development of public services were associated with concerns about damaging family responsibility and increasing dependence (Lewis 1995). Indeed, the basis on which the formal post-war health and welfare system was built was that women would be at home to run the household and provide family care. As demographic and workplace changes mean there are decreasing numbers of women available to offer such community and family care, the rallying cries of carers associations and feminists have meant that the work of unwaged carers has become a matter of increasing significance to paid providers of health care, policy makers and academics (Twigg & Atkin 1994). With this increase in attention to the labour of carers has come the proliferation in the terms used to describe them. Groups tend to refer to themselves as 'carers', whereas legislation, literature, surveys and reports use different terms including family care, household care, community care, informal carers, lay carers, domestic labour, unpaid care and, the term I shall predominantly use in this chapter, unwaged carers. Each of these terms tells a particular story about who is using the term and reveals something about why unwaged care has remained so invisible and so poorly understood for so long.

It seems appropriate to start with the terminology of 'carers' themselves. It was less than 40 years ago, in 1963, that Mary Webster gave up her Congregational Ministry to look after elderly, sick parents. Having realised that her private problem was also a public issue, Webster organised a meeting at the House of Commons. In 1965 as the result of the meeting, the National Council for the Single Woman and Her Dependants was formed 'and the carers' movement can be said to have begun' (Kohner 1993: 5). The name of the Council sounds as though it comes from the nineteenth century, and it was for white, middle-class, professional women, even though it was formed during the relatively radical times of the 1960s. It was only in 1982 that the movement became slightly more embracing, being renamed the National Council for Carers and their Elderly Dependents. In 1988, the Council joined with the Association of Carers (founded in 1981 to focus more specifically on the broader burden of caring, including its costs), to become the Carers National Association, a lobbying group and support system (Kohner 1993).

Although it took years for carers to develop a collective voice of their own, carer support groups have now become significant in their own right, with a network across the country. Yet, despite the campaigning and practical work of these groups, there remain thousands of people who do not know about them or would not recognise themselves as belonging. It was not until 1990 that McCalman, (McCalman 1990) published a report on 'The forgotten people: carers in three minority ethnic communities in Southwark' describing the tasks, difficulties and situation of carers in Afro-Caribbean, Asian and Vietnamese/Chinese communities. In 1993 Aldridge and Becker were among the first to draw attention to the thousands of children who bear a heavy responsibility of care for an adult (Aldridge & Becker 1993).

The danger in writing about those who might describe themselves as 'carers' is that any reference to carers' 'stronger voice' (Kohner 1993) suggests a coherence and agreement among the millions involved, which does not exist. 'Carers' cannot be regarded as a 'sector' to be compared with workers of the public sector, the commercial sector and the voluntary sector. They are bound by moral, psychological and social ties which mean they cannot abandon their carework because it is too demanding. As individuals they do not work in the same context as waged carers, they do not have the same support, the same funding, the same choices, the same ability to leave at the end of the day and go home for a rest. Many have to combine this role, often in a different house, with other roles – not only their own paid work but also roles as wife and mother. Furthermore, carers are subject to stringent outside pressures and social expectations – including from those health and social care professionals who do not understand the multiple, unremitting, calls on carers' time and attention.

Feminists have argued that such work remained invisible for so long because it was seen as women's work, natural, to be expected, and hidden within the confines of the home by a society which emphasises status through waged employment. Such domestic labour has many hidden costs which have life consequences for those involved, some of which are explored in the next section. So it is that the history of caring as 'natural' women's work; the heterogeneity of carers of different cultures, ages and expectations; the sense of family and social obligation; and the privacy of the domestic world, contribute to the invisibility of the work of unwaged carers. These factors all mitigate against public recognition of what is involved.

Moving on to other terminologies, it is intriguing to identify what they convey about the way carers are seen within the overall provision of health and welfare and how easy it is to lose sense of individual people who give and receive care. The growing emphasis on 'community care' since the Second World War is becoming not just 'care in the community' but 'care by the community' – a form of family or household care. The reasons given for this are both ideological, that is, care is best delivered at home in familiar surroundings and also, increasingly, for reasons of financial expediency – that is, as a society we can no longer afford the levels of public service previously offered (Parker 1990, Twigg & Atkin 1994). Family care clearly comes from a centuries old, but nonetheless current belief, that 'family' should decide on and hold prime responsibility for the provision of care to members of the family (Stacey 1988). This is combined with the view that family care is 'best' because the intimacy of personal relations means that the person being cared for, is also cared about (Graham 1983, Finch & Groves 1983). If sentimentalism about this view is allowed to creep in, it is easy to forget that 'family' is also where, for a variety of reasons, most violence takes place, whether it is to children, between adults, or to the elderly. Thus any system which is reliant on 'family' must not only cater for those who do not have family, but also for those for whom family care is fundamentally inappropriate. Similarly, while 'household' care can refer to the nuclear family as well as any collection of people who share accommodation, there is no guarantee that householders are suitable supporters of each others care. The bond may be one born of economic need rather than affection, as anyone who has shared a student hall of residence or a flat will know.

Yet if expectations of family care can tend to be inward looking and uncritical, the term lay carers, can, wittingly or unwittingly, be undermining. The term 'lay' carers primarily draws attention to carers responsibilities and skills relative to 'professional' carers. While the term is broadly based and includes friends, neighbours and networks of carers in addition to family, it compares the 'untrained' with professionals who have achieved a formal qualification and are accountable through a code of professional ethics. If the range of knowledge and skills individual lay carers offer are not recognised, it is easy for the term to become pejorative. A slight twist to this terminology is that, of course, professionals are just as likely to have responsibilities as 'lay' carers as the rest of the population.

Analyses of domestic labour may appear to have little to do with 'unwaged' care. Domestic care is usually associated with looking after the family and housework, whereas unwaged care is identified as work with people with some form of disability. Nevertheless, writing on domestic labour has been crucially important in raising the profile of carers and identifying reasons for the invisibility of their work. Derived from feminist analyses of work, domestic labour refers to the maintenance and reproduction work carried out by women in the privacy of home, but which is fundamental to the economy of most societies. Although it was estimated by Laing (1993), that the financial value of the work of informal carers in 1992 was £39 billion, this does not include parents who care for children, or the adult children who offer financial support to their ageing parents. Even with these exclusions the £39 billion (since criticised for overvaluing the carers at £7 per hour) is more than the public and commercial sectors put together. Yet without this unpaid work society could not manage to care for the chronically ill and those who are disabled.

Another commonly used, but whimsical term, is informal care. Informal care is used as a contrast to the care provided by formally accountable sectors – public (or statutory), commercial and voluntary. These sectors are obliged to act within public, company or charity law; explain what they are doing and why to ministers of health, or shareholders or boards of trustees; and offer their accounts for scrutiny. They are 'formal', because they are constituted in a way that makes them open to question from a range of people. All this makes sense. But 'informal' contains overtones of choice, of opting in an out and of light-heartedness. This apparent informality is in contrast to the structural dependence we, as a society, have for 'informal carers' individually and collectively. This makes it odd to use the term 'informal' to refer to millions of people who together form (whether they should or not) the very foundation of health and social care and without whom the national economy would be dramatically altered.

It is because I find the term 'informal care' misleading that I use the phrase unwaged care. Unwaged care encourages us to bring the millions of people on whom we rely for our health into the broader picture of health provision (see Fig. 12.1). Further, it reminds us of the costs carers bear as they alter their lives in ways which have consequences for their own health and welfare, for most informal carers have a strong sense of obligation and duty because of binding personal ties to those they care for.

Like the other terms, unwaged care is not without its problems. The term may imply that the cost of care should be the prime focus for the society and individuals involved, rather than the 'values' of care. Although there has been a long, tense, debate about whether such care should be paid for by society with a wage (Jordan 1990), there is no sign that such a wage will be forthcoming. Yet some people caught up in caring work do receive a benefit, for example an attendance allowance, or small one-off payments from those whom they care for, which means they are not quite 'unpaid'. However, benefits do not constitute a wage which allows carers to build their own future and make their own choices about their carework.

Who cares?

This section examines who becomes counted and who gets excluded from calculations about unwaged carers, what unwaged carers do and the implications of unwaged care for the carers own life.

Fascinating figures or numbing numbers?

If about 3.5 million people need some form of support to manage their daily life in the privacy of their own home, how is the task shared around and what was it that brought this huge hidden workforce to light? In 1985 the General Household Survey (GHS) had included for the first time an interview question which asked respondents whether they looked after or gave special help to anyone 'sick, handicapped or elderly living in the same household, or if they provided 'some regular service or help' to anyone 'sick, handicapped, or elderly' who lived in a different household' (Parker & Lawton 1994: 1). The figures showed that 14% of people aged 16 and over 'were looking after, or providing some regular service for someone who was sick, elderly or handicapped' (Green 1988: 6), suggesting a national figure of around 6 million people who would identify themselves as being involved in some kind of supportive provision to others. At a repeat survey in 1990, the figure was 6.8 million.

These figures caused a furore not only because they suggested that the amount of invisible caring work was much more than had been guessed, but also because they suggested that men made a major contribution. However, while the figures were higher than anticipated, what was more significant was that 1.5 million people were providing an average of 20 hours work a week, with one million providing over 35 hours work a week – nearly a full working week, unpaid. This figure of 1.5 million is astonishing because it is more than the whole NHS workforce.

On analysing the 1985 GHS figures in more detail it became apparent that, as feminist writers had suspected, women take the major burden of heavy caring work and that the male carers were predominantly spouses or looking after the lighter end of caring. Those most likely to provide unwaged care, in descending order, were spouse, relative in joint household; daughter; daughter-in-law; son; other relative and finally non-relative (Walker & Qureshi 1989). A study identified by Parker and Lawton (1994) of 353 mentally handicapped adults in West Yorkshire showed that the main carers were mother 80%; father 9%; sibling 6%; spouse 1% and other relative 4%, again indicating how extensively the heaviest, most time-consuming burden of care is taken up by women. Nevertheless, the analysis and subsequent follow-up work of the 1985 GHS did bring to light men as another group of 'forgotten carers' (Arber & Gilbert 1989).

Parker's reviews in 1985 and 1990 of 'research on informal care' have been crucial in drawing together statistics which help give some idea of the structural input of unwaged carers. Using figures from a range of sources, Parker suggested that there are nearly 6 million 'disabled' adults (over 16) and children in the country. Of these nearly 0.5 million live in special homes or hospitals, while just over 1 million are in the category of least disabled. Parker's final estimate was of between 3.3 and 3.5 million people living in private households and needing support to manage their daily activities. This number will continue to grow as the population ages, being due to plateau out between 2020 and 2040. The detailed analysis of figures on carers also confirmed earlier work which estimated 1.3–1.8 million 'main' carers of disabled adults and children (Parker 1990, Parker & Lawton 1994).

Although estimating the numbers of unwaged carers has been a matter of considerable debate, such work was crucial because it began to quantify the scale of the task unwaged carers undertake. In policy terms it contributed to bringing about the Carers Recognition and Services Act of 1995 – an Act that would never have been passed had the Carers National Association not lobbied with government on the basis of these figures to establish public recognition of the needs of unwaged carers.

Interestingly, the crucial act of refinement and classification, may itself contribute to hiding the extent of what is involved. National employment statistics cover full and part-time work as a means of identifying trends and making appropriate national policy. In focusing on the 1.3–1.8 million who carry out a bulk of hard, unwaged, carework, focus is on the 24% of informal carers who offer over 20 hours work a week – an enormous amount of money if calculated as paid care. However this leaves out the 75% who do not do as much as a half-time, unpaid, job but remain fundamental to community care policies. It also, inevitably, totally ignores the broader aspects of 'health'. We necessarily miss out those from whom we learn about health in the first place – the parent or parents who teach over 11 million under-15-year-olds about food, hygiene, exercise as well as providing shelter and money and the teachers who teach and reinforce foundation knowledge of health pro-motion. At the other end of the life course, older people are crucial to the national network of childminding and the frail elderly look after the frail elderly in systems of mutual support with varying levels of mutual dependence for the management of day-to-day living. Other, younger people, themselves with physical disability may well be acting as a support to an elderly parent. Adults, children, friends and neighbours contribute to health care by the community but for most, like parents, this work is part of a relatively ignored fabric of care.

Unwaged carers are, thus, a very heterogeneous category. Adequately negotiated help for unwaged carers must be able to manage not only diversity in what carers do and 'elements of timing, frequency, urgency, complexity and the amount of time the tasks take' (Parker 1990: 5), but also their relationship with the person they care for, different cultural requirements and the individual needs and expectations of unwaged carers and those they care for. As Twigg and Atkin (1995) identify, most of the support offered to carers is through front-line service providers such as GPs, social workers and community nurses, who have, until now, been there primarily for the person being cared for. It is how these front-line providers negotiate with carers as well as users which deter-mines the access unwaged carers get to other services – which is why it is so crucial that everyone involved in health and social welfare has a sound understanding of the work of unwaged carers.

It is clear that there is no consensus about what is meant by unwaged care and so, even if research methods could identify all the individuals in the privacy of their homes and community who offer some form of 'care', there is no agreement on what to count. It helps to recognise the com-plexity of making this calculation if we think about our own family and friends. We can consider which of those people have someone depending on them for the management of their day-to-day physical and mental health, but also whether they would refer to themselves as carers. Certainly, on an autobiographical note, without the grandparents looking after our children in the school holidays, my sisters and I would have considerable difficulty in managing home and work – a pattern repeated across the country.

What do carers do?

Analytically, distinctions can be made between 'care' in a broad sense of helping with everyday household and financial tasks; psychological support; and 'tending' – the provision of physical care (Walker & Qureshi 1989, Leger 1992). Parker and Lawton (1994) draw on 3061 cared-for people (some carers looked after more than one person), identified through the 1985 GHS to develop a typology of six categories of caring activity based on tasks. The categories shown in Table 12.1 refer to clusters of associated tasks. *Personal care* involves the most intimate caring work such as washing, dressing, bowel evacuation, management of double incontinence; *physical care* includes getting someone in and out of bed, help with walking; *practical help* covers tasks such as preparing meals, shopping, housework and *support* includes assistance with paperwork and keeping company. *Other help* refers to any combination of support, taking out, keeping an eye on and giving medicines.

Table 12.1 Categories of caring.

Category	% Women	% Men	%
1. Personal *and* physical care	67	33	12
2. Personal *not* physical care	74	26	9
3. Physical *not* personal care	50	50	8
4. Practical help *and* support	60	40	55
5. Practical help only	50	50	8
6. Other help	60	40	14
Base (100%)			3032

Source: Parker, G. & Lawton, D. (1994) *Different Types of Care, Different Types of Carer.* Adapted from pp. 14, 94–7.

In these categories, women were most likely to be involved in the first two (the more intimate forms of tending), while male carers were more likely to be providing categories 3 and 5 – physical not personal care and practical help only. Furthermore, the oldest carers, i.e. over 66, represented 22% of carers in the first category (which is both intimate and often 'heavy'), compared with only 15% in the other categories. An additional, crucial finding, is the age of those cared for. Those below the age of 65 are over-represented in the first two 'heavier' caring categories involving personal care, whereas those 66 and over are more likely to be in receipt of practical, rather than personal forms of care. The importance of this is that it shows that older people are able to maintain high degrees of independence as it is the practical, domestic tasks with which they need most help. A more surprising finding is that the majority of those who most needed intensive informal care (i.e. personal and physical care) were under 65. This has huge implications in terms of the length of time such unwaged care must be sustained for each person receiving it and says much about the desperate need for respite care (Warner 1994, Parker & Lawton 1994).

In looking at unwaged carers' tasks, it is important to look at not only who carries out the tasks, but the forms of dependence that make them necessary. For some unwaged carers support is to a demented person whose physical abilities are impeded by their mental state with the result that the person needs to be fed, cleaned, dressed, entertained and watched over. Disruptive behaviour may have a greater impact on other members of the household than physical disabilities which need constant support.

'...I have 4 children, one who is severely mentally handicapped. He causes such havoc in the house that it is a strain not just on my husband and myself, but also to the other children as well. He has a younger brother who has been punished since he was born, shall we say from his brother. So it is essential that he goes out of the home.'

(Warner 1994: 46)

While severity of disability must be taken into account, as Parker and Lawton (1994) importantly point out, this does not tell us much about what people 'need'. Those who receive help from unwaged carers may do so because they are in inappropriate housing with inappropriate facilities for washing, shopping (telephone shopping could make a big difference) and cooking, and not enough money to sustain themselves. In many circumstances, if these were available in the right kinds of forms, the demand on unwaged carers could be reduced and the independence of the disabled person increased. This brings us back to the question posed at the beginning of the chapter about whether, as a society, we should redress the balance of responsibilities expected of unwaged carers and replace it with policies which offer a stronger collective, rather than individual, response.

Contributions, implications and support

Costs to unwaged carers can be physical, emotional, financial and social, showing themselves through restricted social opportunities (20% of a sample of unwaged carers 'never get a break' – Carers National Association 1992); reduced employment opportunities; increased expenditure and physical and emotional strain. Two authors from the Centre for Health Economics at York noted:

> 'From an economic perspective it is important to assess the deploy-ment of the informal care resource, as with any other resource, to ensure the maximization of the social benefit generated by these scarce resources.'   (Smith & Wright 1994: 138)

While the distant, feelingless tone of the York paper could hardly con-trast more with the commitment of Jimmy or the desperation of the mother with the disruptive mentally handicapped child, it is intended to help support unwaged carers in their choices. It does so by attempting to assess the negative consequences of caring against the more positive aspects of 'feelings experienced and satisfaction gained' (Smith & Wright 1994: 139), noting that 'the carer may be expected to assess the relative costs and benefits of these options in making decisions'. Such rational analysis may have little to contribute to the carer identified by Twigg and Atkin as Ms Myers, but it is a measure of how far the consequences of unwaged care have penetrated into policy analysis. Ms Myers was a single unemployed woman in her thirties looking after her mother with severe dementia and 'seemed in a permanent state of crisis, mesmerised by her situation and with no emotional energy left to take control of her own chaotic finances' (Twigg & Atkin 1994: 11).

The financial consequences of caring have begun to be outlined (Glendinning 1992). Additional analysis indicates that even where unwaged carers do have paid employment it tends to be in low paid jobs which best fit the demands of their unwaged carework. Thus carers not only bear increased expense through heating, lighting and house-keeping, but suffer loss of higher level income and lose the ability to contribute to the pension that will help them in their own retirement. Since, as a society we are increasingly moving toward some form of additional social insurance to contribute to care in old age (Health Committee 1996, Joseph Rowntree Foundation 1996, Laing 1993), unwaged carers may become even more disadvantaged, losing the ability to contribute to two sets of future benefit. Other legacies of caring include consequences to psychological, social and physical health, which while not affecting everyone, may leave some carers in difficulties after the person they are caring for dies or moves into a home:

> '... I never see anybody from one end of the week to the other really ... I suppose probably that is why I get so depressed every now and again that is how it affects me ... it would have helped to have a break ... we were tied to the house all the time ... I would go to the shop each day

for a few bits and do my weekly shopping and that was my most time out of the house.' (McLaughlin & Ritchie 1994: 246)

Here the carer has lost social contacts over the years and, now in need of distraction and support herself, has no-one to help. Yet Smith and Wright (1994) suggest the negative consequences are sometimes over-emphasised because they underestimate the alternatives. They give examples of the alternatives such as the 'burden of care' associated with the guilt of having a loved one in a residential home, travel time and the expense of contributing to different forms of care.

Support for carers

Policy makers are becoming increasingly aware of the extent and significance of the work of unwaged carers. The 1988 Griffiths Report (DHSS 1988) proposed that action be taken to assess informal carers' needs and was a sign that policy makers recognised that something needed to be done. This report led to the 1989 White Paper 'Caring for People'and contributed to the 1990 National Health Service and Community Care Act. The Carers Recognition and Services Act was passed in 1996 following strong lobbying from the Carers National Association, research from the General Household Survey showing the significance of the issues on a national basis and Government recognition of the need for radical change in community and acute care services The 1996 Act was primarily aimed at the 1.5 million carers working over 20 hours a week, including the 1 million who provide care for over 35 hours a week. It entitled carers to a needs assessment of their own, separate to that of the 'user', encouraging (with no extra budget) provision that might include domiciliary and day services, short-stay respite and residential care.

While it is possible to interpret this Act as an important move in public recognition of the worth of unwaged carers, it should not be mis-interpreted. Questions still remain as to whether the support covers all those who need it and whether it is adequate for those who have been identified as in need. Evaluations of local authority provision for both users and carers remain mixed (Smith *et al.* 1993, Lewis & Glennerster 1996). The growth of carers groups, themselves promoted by local authorities, help the profile of unwaged carers, but many carers find themselves unable to make the arrangements necessary to allow them to attend for support, even if they know, or care about them.

Unwaged carers are in a middle ground. They work between users, who are in theory the focus of attention, and the policies of the formal sectors. Both users and the sectors depend on the work of unwaged carers while at least in part contributing to the social and moral forces which anticipate that unwaged carers will want to, or should, provide for those close to them. Meantime, the heterogeneous population of unwaged carers have highly differentiated experiences of the value and cost of carework in their lives.

Unwaged carers and the wider social context

As unwaged carers were invisible for so many years, so the inter-connections between unwaged carers and other providers of health services were ignored. Similarly, the interdependence of individual service users and unwaged carers was lost within the overall context of health provision. This partial picture can only be amended by looking at the interconnections of individual citizens, unwaged carers and provision in public, voluntary and commercial sectors.

Unwaged carers are fundamental to the working of the public, commercial and voluntary sectors, but are also consumers of the welfare provided by them. In recognising this mutual dependence between substantive groups, the significance of the reciprocity involved in carework both at a structural level and at an individual level can be identified. Caregivers can be involved in multiple ways. An individual may be an unwaged (domestic) carer, part of the commercial sector (occasional paid or agency work), the public sector (employed in the primary or secondary services) and involved in voluntary work (helping through a range of community groups from Samaritans to Childline to local fund-raising and self help). However, in taking account of this structural and individual interdependence, it is still easy to lose a sense of the partici-pation and reciprocity of those who give and 'receive' tending care. The informed, diligent carer of a child with chronic asthma, will still use health services himself when he gets arthritis. To define him either as a patient or a carer is to misconstrue the totality of his interconnections with health services. Similarly, to define a doctor, who happens to have diabetes but who also offers a session free to a homeless drop-in centre and supports her dependent mother merely as a user, or a volunteer, or a professional carer, or an unwaged carer diminishes the interdependence of all these roles. It also misconstrues the part her mother has played in health, when, formerly, she was the unwaged carer to a growing daughter. Although current health measures include levels of 'dependence' as criteria for a range of purposes, including staff allocation, all of us 'depend' on each other, and on various forms of 'unwaged care' for multiple functions of everyday living. For these reasons it is important for us to develop an understanding of the interdependence of individuals in society.

In addition to missing out the central contribution of unwaged carers, for many years the interconnections between the public, commercial and voluntary systems of health delivery were also lost. Professionals and academics concentrated their attention on understanding and developing the detail of the group or sector with whom they were most involved. In the late 1980s and 1990s, as pressure on the public services increased, so an understanding of how all the different forms of health delivery work together with unwaged carers provoked new interest.

Citizens: unwaged carers and the health care diamond

The 'health care diamond' (Fig. 12.1), considerably adapted from Pijl's 'welfare diamond' (Pijl 1994) is a visual image of how individuals and health sectors interconnect. The individual citizens form the focus in the centre. Each citizen is not merely a 'recipient' of care, but an active user, for the most part negotiating their own care and, at some stage in their life, usually giving care to others. There are times in our lives when all of us are recipients of care, but for many it is a relatively small part of our middle years which carry on in other ways, offering emotional, financial and physical support to others. Thus, the 'citizen' in the middle, is all of us as individuals. It suggests our interdependence with others, but also suggests the fluidity between the citizen in the middle and the different categories on the outside points of the diamond. Nurses, doctors, social workers, home helps, paid carers, teachers, nutritionists, opticians,

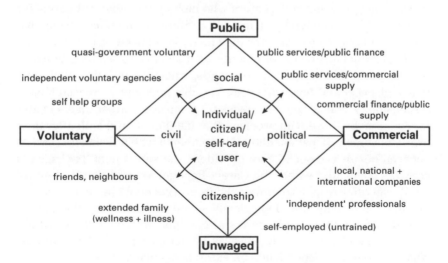

Fig. 12.1 Health care Diamond. James (1995), adapted from Pijl's 'Welfare Diamond' in *Payments in Care*, 1994.

dentists, physiotherapists, domestics and so on, that is millions of us, may be a 'patient', or use the pharmacist for over-the-counter drugs, or be part of a self-help group for a chronic illness such as depression, without withdrawing support to others. This continuing mutuality means that there are always interconnections between us as individual citizens and the sectors with whom we not only negotiate, but may be a part of.

The diamond suggests a range of nuances within and between the groups that contribute to health. For example, what is referred to in the health care diamond as the commercial sector includes independent health professionals, complementary therapists and paid carers (Leat & Gay 1987), as well as established residential care chains and private hospitals. With these nuances the complexity surrounding 'unwaged' care is, inevitably, immensely varied. These variations have, as some of the unwaged carer quotes suggest, real consequences, with the impact of a particular constellation of care being dramatic for those involved. For example, one of the issues facing unwaged carers is that nearly all employers ask for relevant work experience and for a reference from a recent employer. An unwaged carer may be able to show the first of these, but not the second. Thus variation in response to need may offer greater flexibility, but is also harder to understand, negotiate and research.

There are also other reasons for placing unwaged carers within the broader picture of health provision, the prime one of which is to remind us that a change in one sector is likely to cause a change for others. If public and commercial sectors send people home quickly after oper-ations (because 'home' is a better place to convalesce and because it saves money) it is unwaged carers who pick up the labour of caring for someone still debilitated by an operation. Similarly, if policies mean that access to public sector care for the elderly is reduced or becomes sub-ject to personal insurance, or requires an individual to sell their house, it is likely to be families, or close friends, who pick up additional emo-tional, physical and financial costs. Yet, this policy of increased 'family responsibility' will be seen as a measure of success, rather than a matter for concern, by those who proclaim that families should look after their own. Conversely, if 'patient choice' is combined with a 'seamless service' between health and social care providers, the subsequent 'packages of care' (as advocated within the Carers Recognition and Services Act of 1995), can offer respite to unwaged carers. This could be seen as a long overdue, financially and ideologically sound development which facili-tates the ability of unwaged carers to continue with a vitally necessary task. Alternately, it could be seen as an inappropriate additional cost which encourages dependence on external agencies.

Placing the millions of individuals who contribute to unwaged care, however broadly or narrowly unwaged care is defined, within a health care diamond is not without controversy. To make unwaged carers the base of the diamond is to show how fundamental their work is to the health and welfare of the country. The danger is that it also somehow implies that all the millions of individuals are included on the same basis as other health and welfare workers, the paid health carers who work as part of teams, who can have time off sick and who take annual leave. Nevertheless, the health care diamond does offer a way of beginning to take account of the reciprocity and interdependence of unwaged carers with other health and social care providers and also of thinking about the relationship and interdependence between unwaged carers and those whom they support. A major question remains unresolved – how best to identify, analyse and form policy associated with unwaged carers. Should unwaged carers be considered as a whole, a form of sector, thus taking full account of their collective contribution to the health and welfare of the country, or should the millions of different individuals be recognised as being different to each other, albeit with some elements in common? This question has implications at three levels – individual, organisational and societal – which require us to:

- think through the life consequences for individual unwaged carers
- understand the impact on unwaged carers of change in health delivery
- analyse the implications of societal expectations of 'family responsibility'.

The last of these is the one that has an impact on all of us. Everyone needs to consider how much we could or should contribute to the care of parents, friends, siblings, children and neighbours in terms of physical, emotional, social and financial support. This means considering whether, as individuals we should think of ourselves as part of a major national caring team, a kind of collective structural support, or whether we should think of ourselves as lone individual agents. Each of these has different implications for privacy, rights and expectations. In either case unwaged carers (who may also be paid carers) are different to the myriad of other forms of health worker while remaining subject to the consequences of national policies on a day-to-day basis.

Conclusions

The seventeenth century poetry of John Donne quoted at the beginning of this chapter movingly captures our interdependence on each other. More than that, he visits a collective and also much more private world, in which we are all part of a whole. If one of us is lost, we are all reduced, and the death of one of us is the partial death of all of us: 'ask not for whom the bell tolls, it tolls for thee'. In his terms, there is no separation of individual and society.

Exploring the connections between the millions of individuals involved in unwaged care and the social requirement that this care be provided is part of an unending sociological exploration of the relation between the individual and society. The search for an understanding of these connections between individual and society invites us to examine the present and the future with growing localisation, globalisation and technology – all with an impact on how health and ill health is managed. Demographic trends, traditional 'family' mores, women's place, the melding of public and private worlds (for example through home working, telephone shopping, banking, the Internet) and technological developments all herald change in the relations between individuals and society and thereby the ideologies, planning and delivery of health services. Greater emphasis on primary care, self-care, self and family provision and prevention; divisions between 'health care' and 'social care'; deregulation of over-the-counter remedies for self treatment; telemedicine; and rapid hospital discharge all have implications not only for the patients, but also for unwaged carers and their relations with the broader health context. At sociological and social policy levels, the emphasis on choice of individuals as agents and on family responsibility is at odds with more collective, structural approaches which involve greater state intervention.

References

Aldridge, J. & Becker, S. (1993) *Children Who Care: Inside the World of Young Carers*. Department of Social Sciences, Loughborough University.

Arber, S. & Gilbert, N. (1989) Men: the forgotten carers. *Sociology*, **23**, 111–18.

Carers National Association (1992) *Speak Up, Speak Out*. Chilworth Mews, London.

DHSS (Department of Health and Social Security) (1988) *Community Care: Agenda for Action*. HMSO, London.

Finch, J. & Groves, D. (1983) *A Labour of Love: Women, Work and Caring*. Routledge, London.

Glendinning, C. (1992) *The Costs of Informal Care*. SPRU, York.

Graham, H. (1983) Caring: a labour of love. In: *Labour of Love: Women, Work and Caring* (eds J. Finch & D. Groves). Routledge, London.

Green, H. (1988) Informal carers. *General Household Survey 1985*. HMSO, London.

Health Committee (1996) *Long-term Care: Future Provision and Funding*, HC 59-1. HMSO, London.

Jordan, B. (1990) *Value for Caring: Recognising Unpaid Carers*. Kings Fund, London.

Joseph Rowntree Foundation Inquiry (1996) *Meeting the Costs of Continuing Care: Report and Recommendations*. Joseph Rowntree Foundation, York.

Kohner, N. (1993) *A Stronger Voice: The Achievements of the Carers' movement 1963–1993*. Carers National Association, Glasshouse Yard, London.

Laing, W. (1993) *Financing Long-term Care: The Crucial Debatge*. Age Concern, London.

Leat, D. & Gay, P. (1987) *Paying for Care: A Study of Policy and Practice in Paid Care Schemes*. Policy Studies Institute, London.

Leger, F.S. (1992) Informal welfare: policy debate and sociological reality. *Social Policy Review*, **4**.

Lewis, J. (1995) Family provision of health and welfare in the mixed economy of care in the late nineteenth and twentieth centuries. *Social History of Medicine*, **1**, 1–16.

Lewis, J. & Glennerster, H. (1996) *Implementing the New Community Care*. Open University Press, Buckingham.

McCalman, J.A. (1990) *The Forgotten People: Carers in Three Minority Ethnic Communities in Southwark*. King's Fund Centre with Help the Aged, London.

McLaughlin, E. & Ritchie, J. (1994) Legacies of caring: the experiences and circumstances of ex-carers. *Health and Social Care in the Community*, **2**, 241–53.

Parker, G. (1990) *With Due Care and Attention: A Review of Research on Informal Care* (2nd edn). Family Policies Study Centre, London.

Parker, G. & Lawton, D. (1994) *Different Types of Care. Different Types of Carer: Evidence from the GHS*. HMSO, London.

Pijl, M. (1994) When private care goes public. In: *Payments for Care: A Comparative Overview* (eds A. Evers, M. Pijl & C. Ungerson). Avebury, Aldershot.

Smith, K. & Wright, K. (1994) Informal care and economic appraisal: a discussion of possible methodological approaches. *Health Economics*, **3**, 137–48.

Smith, R., Gaster, L., Harrison, L., Martin, L., Means, R. & Thistlethwaite, P. (1993) *Working Together for Better Community Care*. SAUS, Bristol.

Stacey, M. (1988) *The Sociology of Health and Healing*. Unwin Hyman, London.

Twigg, J. & Atkin, K. (1994) *Carers Perceived: Policy and Practice in Informal Care*. Open University Press, Buckingham.

Twigg, J. & Atkin, K. (1995) Carers and services: factors mediating service provision. *Journal of Social Policy*, **24**, 5–30.

Walker, A. & Qureshi, H. (1989) *The Caring Relationship*. Macmillan, Basingstoke.

Warner, N. (1994) *Community Care: Just a Fairy Tale?* University of Kent, Canterbury.

Index